D0892046

ADVOCACY AND EMPOWERMENT

ADVOCACY AND EMPOWERMENT
Mental Health Care in the Community

Stephen M. Rose and Bruce L. Black

ROUTLEDGE & KEGAN PA~~~
BOSTON, LONDON AND H~

To
Dale Selwyn

First published in 1985
by Routledge & Kegan Paul plc

9 Park Street, Boston, Mass. 02108, USA

14 Leicester Square, London WC2H 7PH, England and

Broadway House, Newtown Road,
Henley on Thames, Oxon RG9 1EN, England

Set in Times, 10 on 12 pt
by Inforum Ltd, Portsmouth
and printed in Great Britain
by Billings and Sons Ltd,
Worcester

Library of Congress Cataloging in Publication Data

Rose, Stephen M.
  Advocacy and empowerment.

  Bibliography: p.
  1. Mental health services—United States.   2. Mentally
ill—Rehabilitation—United States.   3. Mental health
policy—United States.   4. Mental health laws—United
States.   I. Black, Bruce.   II. Title. [DNLM: 1. After
Care.   2. Community Mental Health Service.   3. Patient
Advocacy. WM 29 R797a]
  RA790.6.R66   1985   *362.2'0973*   *85–1802*

ISBN 0–7100–9963–0

Contents

Acknowledgments

Most of the work which led to the creation of this book was done through the Mental Health Project at the School of Social Welfare (at the State University of New York at Stony Brook) and at the Sayville Project Community Support Systems program. Many people, both staff and students, were involved in contributing to our efforts in building and guiding a critical, theoretically informed practice through the Mental Health Project and Sayville Project programs. We would especially like to mention a number of staff people whose creativity and commitment were of particular significance to us: from the NIMH/Mental Health Project, Donna Chaglasian, Ettie Taichman, Judith Jones, Peggy Brennan, Polly Purvis; and, from the Sayville Project, Paul Sivak, David Finke, Marie Chandick, Arlene Schwartz, Diane Achenbach Zatorski, Paul Stein, David Walsh. Each of these individuals went well beyond the specific jobs they held to engage actively in the overall purpose – to create and implement an advocacy/ empowerment orientation to practice.

Dale Selwyn, a wonderful friend and colleague on the Mental Health Project, died in July 1984. Dale meant a great deal to us: as a colleague, she brought a finely honed intelligence to her work and ours; a sense of unrelenting commitment both to our clients and to our practice principles; and a warm loving sense of humor which sustained us all. We want to dedicate this book to her as a way of saying 'Thank you.'

Diane M. Johnson, our colleague from the Legal Advocacy and Organizing Project, deserves special mention. She brought to the task of critical review of the manuscript the exact combination of theoretical understanding and editorial acumen that earlier versions required. Without her disciplined and caring input, we could not have produced the work we wanted. We are deeply appreciative of her skill and commitment to the work.

We also want to thank a number of people with whom we met through contact with various funding agencies. We want to thank these individuals for their positive contribution to the growth and development of our Project: Dr Marta Sotomayor from the National Institute of Mental Health, along with Dr Milton Wittman and Dr Neilson Smith, gave us incise criticism and suggestions which allowed our direct service program to function more effectively and our graduate student training program to be more systematic; Hagop Mashikian, M.D., and John Iafrate, M.D., Regional Directors of the Long Island Region, New York State Office of Mental Health, Elmer Bertsch, Deputy Director, and Gloria Logsdon, Program Analyst, were all willing to support and sustain a program that incurred the wrath of numerous and powerful mental health agencies. The normal 'gatekeeping' activities of Projects funded through grants and contracts were expanded and our work enhanced through the interactions we had with these people. We also want to thank the Veatch Program of the North Shore Unitarian Society for funding us to do our legal and legislative advocacy work, and to express our appreciation to two state legislators, Paul Harenberg and Robert Wertz, who gave us valuable insight and advice, without partisan concern, that allowed us to promote just and effective legislation.

And we want to thank the numerous former patients who let us into their lives, sometimes at risk to themselves from their landlords or workers from conventional service agencies. As we write this note of gratitude, a series of poignant moments with individuals come flooding to memory, a reflection of the emotional intensity that characterized this Project, its commitment to human dignity, and its struggle for social change.

We would like to think that this book honors Dale, our colleagues, and the shared experience with students and ex-patients. For all that contributes to maintaining the fight against oppression and domination, we owe you our deep thanks. For errors and ambiguities, we are solely responsible and we apologize.

Stephen M. Rose

November 1984   Stony Brook, New York

Introduction

Deinstitutionalization, as a social policy, has had a complex and confusing history. We will try to unravel much of the complexity and decipher a good deal of the mystification surrounding this policy in order to develop a clear and coherent framework for creating and sustaining a positive and systematic practice in the area of mental health after-care. We take it for granted that a coherent theory of practice must be a conscious correlate of a larger theory that addresses the social world in which that practice will occur. It is this belief that gives rise to our organizing rationale for this book. As you can see from the Table of Contents, the first section of the book is theoretical – our effort to explain the social world of working in mental health after-care. Initially, we provide a brief analysis of deinstitutionalization as a social policy, looking carefully at who it was intended to serve and who in fact has benefited from its existence. Along the way, we will identify several essential contradictions within the policy and its political economic context that have functioned as determinants of the policy throughout its history. Next there is an effort to create what we call a 'problem-definition' level of theory: how are we to look at the reality of former patients' lives? How we perceive that reality will ultimately inform our intervention into it (Kuhn, 1962), and therein lies our effort at articulating our theory of practice, the purpose of Chapter 2. The first section concludes with a chapter on social action strategy, the larger design for implementing our advocacy/empowerment approach to practice.

One of the more complex problems encountered in examining deinstitutionalization is differentiating between the availability or accessability of services and the appropriateness of them, in those cases where services do exist. One way of looking into this issue is historical review, but even that is problematic. Consensus exists, together with plentiful documentation, about the fact that after-care services were rarely, if ever, in place when the process of wholesale discharge of patients from state psychiatric hospitals began. While most adherents of mental health ideology claim that deinstitutionalization began with federal intervention into mental health policy and planning in 1963, or with the widespread use of psychotropic drugs just prior to that time, the process of discharging patients and emptying beds began well before that, in 1955. That same year, President Eisenhower appointed the Joint Commission on Mental Illness and Mental Health to assess the situation in The United States and to recommend a policy direction.

The year 1963 marks the first time the federal government articulated a nationwide social policy about mental health services, an area previously managed by state government and/or counties. From the introduction of Community Mental Health Center legislation in 1963 through to the late 1970s, the discharging process escalated, eventually lowering the number of occupied inpatient beds in state and county psychiatric hospitals by more than 65 per cent. The growth of after-care services followed much more slowly, in part because the federally funded Community Mental Health Centers (CMHC) were supposed to provide a full array of after-care services but did not do so. While former patients certainly knew that little or nothing existed to serve them, it took quite a while for professionals and planners to grasp that fact adequately. As you will see from what follows in this introduction, we believe the advent of mental health after-care as a particular area of practice was approximately 1975, a time when community outrage coupled with rapidly advancing recidivism rates combined economic and political pressures to push for a more adequately construed definition of what needed to be done.

At the federal level, as evidenced by a Report to the Congress by the Comptroller General, entitled *Returning the Mentally Disabled to the Community: Government Needs to do More* (1977), and by the report of The President's Commission on Mental Health (1978), a clear consciousness existed about the neglect shown to former patients, particularly those described as 'chronically mentally ill.' The Mental Health Systems Act of 1980 targeted this group as a top priority, stating that thousands of such people 'receive deplorably inadequate assistance' (President's Commission, 1978, p. vii).

In the State of New York, which housed over 90,000 people in its public mental hospitals in 1955, critical examination of the after-care scene was provided by State legislative reports in 1975: the Legislative Commission on Expenditure Review (LCER), in its study, *Patients Released from State Psychiatric Centers*, documented the decrease in inpatient beds from the 90,000+ figure in 1955 to 61,889 in 1970 to 33,684 in 1975 (LCER, 1975, p. S–3). The New York State Assembly Joint Committee to Study the Department of Mental Hygiene, which convened in June 1975, described the inadequacy of services not only in New York, but in several other states which they examined (NYS Assembly Joint Committee, 1976). The Legislative Commission also documented a fact common to more than New York – even though a significantly greater number than 50 per cent of the inpatient beds had been emptied by 1973–4, only 6.5 per cent of state hospital resources were reallocated from institutional settings to outpatient care (LCER, 1975, p. 39). Doctor James Prevost, then Commissioner of the New York State Department of Mental Hygiene, in a report to the Governor for 1978, stated, 'Since 1975, the state has stepped up its efforts to support the development and expansion of community-based services . . .' (Prevost, 1978, p. 6).

The matter of creating community-based services was seen as equivalent to providing appropriate services. The criteria for what constituted 'appropriate' generally went unexplored. Psychiatric domination of mental health services was carried over from institutional care to community based care in the federally funded CMHCs. They were mandated to provide 'five essential services', all clinical in approach, except for consultation and education, a service designed to inform community agencies and institutions about psychiatric intervention and develop referral procedures. 'C & E' as it came to be called, was often little more than a marketing mechanism for psychiatric intervention. The pattern of psychiatric control continuing into community-based programs meant that the shift from hospital-based care to community-based care was in reality only a shift in the locus (as opposed to the focus) of the mental health service delivery system without a concomitant shift in approach to the redefining of, and therefore intervening into, problem situations.

With a medicalized approach to problem definition uncritically in control, psychiatrically defined services were presumed to be as 'appropriate' to clients' needs in the community as they were in the hospital. This transfer of hegemony and legitimation 'depoliticized' the issues and continued the focus of concern on patterns of service delivery rather than on redefining an entire new set of needs that former patients incur as a result of being either de- or reinstitutionalized into community settings. We believe that prevailing views are becoming cloudy in terms of after-care, and questions are arising about what criteria in fact are best for determining what is 'appropriate'. But before moving into this discussion, we want to pursue our retrospective overview.

Mental health after-care, as a concentrated area for policy development, occurred some twenty years after the practice of massive discharging began. While President Kennedy's 'bold new approach' speech of 1963 is generally thought to be the introduction of federal involvement in mental health care, and the subsequent Mental Health Centers Act is hailed as the first piece of progressive legislation in the reform of mental health service delivery, we have dated the advent of mental health after-care in 1975. Our reasons for choosing this later date reflect a belief that change from institutional psychiatry to community-based care can best be understood from an economic rather than mental health framework. By 1975 the goal of reducing state hospital inpatient populations had been reached: the reduction in the number of inpatients in public mental hospitals went from 559,000 in 1955 to approximately 215,000 by 30 June 1974, a reduction of 57 per cent (Comptroller General, 1977, p. 8). In a five state study conducted by the Comptroller General of the United States, there was a 65 per cent reduction between 1963–74. In New York the reduction between 1965–75 was from 84,859 to 33,885, approximately 60 per cent (NYS Assembly Joint Committee, 1976). By 1980, the number had dropped even further, to 24,000 (New York State Office of Mental Health, Five Year plan for 1981, p. 13).

The problems that emerged, in the face of the apparent success (depopulation of state hospitals) of the deinstitutionalization movement were twofold: grossly inadequate services were all that existed in most of the communities that received the discharged patients, and rehospitalization rates began to accelerate, thus increasing a portion of the expenditures which states had hoped would stabilize or drop from decreasing inpatient populations. As inpatients, whatever care was available was the exclusive domain of the hospital – the total institution, as Goffman so aptly described it (Goffman, 1961). Upon release, however, neither communities nor agencies had the capacity to deliver comprehensive services. The chaos that emerged was documented by the Comptroller General:

> Deinstitutionalization has not received the full and well-coordinated support of many State and local agencies administering programs that serve or can serve the mentally disabled. Moreover, agencies serving population groups that do or could include the mentally disabled have not included deinstitutionalization of the mentally disabled in their program plans nor have they made it a specific operating objective or priority. Furthermore, they have not provided financial or other support needed to help mentally disabled persons (1) avoid unnecessary admission or readmission to public institutions, (2) leave such facilities, or (3) receive appropriate help in communities. (Comptroller General, 1977, p. 24)

Furthermore, while state psychiatric facilities were depositing upwards of 65 per cent of their inpatients in underserviced communities, they were not concomitantly reallocating their budgets so that state mental health dollars followed patients from facility to community. As noted above, in New York the percentage of total facility budgets directed to out-patient care in 1974 was only 6.5, an increase of 63 per cent from the previous year (LCER, 1975, p. 38).

By 1975 recidivism in New York, as measured by the number of readmissions to state facilities, had risen from 12,514 in 1965 to 21,591 (NYS Assembly Joint Committee, 1976, p. 17). The data collected by the Legislative Commission found that 17,501 people were readmitted to New York State psychiatric hospitals between April 1974 and March 1975. By 1975, over 63 per cent of all admissions to mental hospitals in New York were readmissions. The growing parade between hospitals and communities had increased elsewhere as well, leading to a new term in conventional psychiatric parlance – 'the revolving door' patient. According to the Report of the Comptroller General, the problem was nationwide in scope:

> Readmissions account for an increasingly large proportion of admissions to public mental hospitals. In 1969, 47 per cent of those entering public mental hospitals had been in such facilities before, but by 1972, the percentage had increased to about 54 per cent. (Comptroller General, 1977, p. 22)

The role of the federal government in stimulating deinstitutionalization accelerated in 1975, taking the form of both legislative and federal court initiatives. Through several bills signed into law, the federal government continued to encourage or induce states to shift from institutional to community mental health patterns of service delivery and to increase the focus on after-care. The 1975 amendments to the Community Mental Health Centers Act stressed after-care as a salient priority: they added seven new services, including housing, and mandated follow-up care for former patients discharged into their catchment areas. The Special Health Revenue Sharing Act of 1975 required states to create and implement a plan which would try to eradicate inappropriate placements in institutions, to develop alternative community-based services, and to push for more careful planning for post-discharge services. In the area of mental retardation a similar process occurred with the passage of the Developmentally Disabled Assistance and Bill of Rights Act. By 1975 The Department of Health, Education and Welfare (now known as the Department of Health and Human Services) had also discovered that while its Medicaid program had directly stimulated deinstitutionalization, it had a confining influence as well – it promoted placement of the mentally disabled in nursing homes and intermediate care facilities. Title XX also came into being in 1975 mandating delivery of social services to Supplemental Security Income (SSI) recipients directed toward maintaining self-sufficiency and providing community-based care (Comptroller General, 1977, pp. 218–19).

The judicial branch of government also played an active supporting role. Three major lawsuits were determined in 1975, each of which involved a decision by a Federal Court, and each of which spurred deinstitutionalization as a judicial mandate. The effect of these decisions was to add a legal rationale to the already existing impetus to decrease state hospital beds. In a case popularly known as the 'Willowbrook Consent Decree' (but actually named New York State Association for Retarded Children v. Carey), a U.S. District Court supported the right of mentally retarded residents to 'treatment in the least restrictive setting.' It also specified that standards for care be established in the context of the new meaning of 'least restrictive setting,' that the inpatient population be reduced significantly, that community placements be created and implemented, and that funds be sought from the legislature to accomplish the objectives stipulated (Comptroller General, 1977, p. 219). This decision reaffirmed the principle of least restrictive setting established three years earlier, in the 1972 US District Court decision in the Wyatt v. Stickney case. This case was a class action lawsuit brought against the state mental health system in

Alabama and resulted in the application of constitutional law to mental patients' rights and to constitutionally determined standards for inpatient care, requiring the hospital to prove that no other less restrictive settings were feasible for each person institutionalized (Comptroller General, 1977, p. 213).

Legal intervention into mental health policy and practice received an even greater impetus in another 1975 decision. In O'Connor v. Donaldson, the U.S. Supreme Court entered the realm of mental health policy-making, asserting that states cannot confine people in mental hospitals who are not dangerous and who are capable of surviving safely alone or with others in the community. The Court did not act on the right to treatment issue, a stance that had been asserted in both the US District Court and the Court of Appeals. The matter of 'right to treatment' basically states that mental hospitals cannot continuously confine people without demonstrating that such treatments exist which will assist people in alleviating their mental illness (Comptroller General, 1977, p. 220).

Another major case was settled during 1975; Dixon v. Weinberger, in a manner similar to the Willowbrook case, determined that involuntarily committed patients at St Elizabeth's Hospital in Washington, D.C. have a right to placement in the least restrictive setting, and that alternative facilities to the hospital must be created for those patients who do not require confinement. In contrast to Wyatt and Donaldson, where the decisions affirm the rights of patients and protect them from infringement by the states, Dixon established that states must not only refrain from infringement, but must redress that situation by providing alternative settings and services appropriate to the person's needs (Comptroller General, 1977, p. 220).

It is interesting to note the political climate in which the decisions mentioned occurred: depopulating state hospitals had been underway for about twenty years; criticism of the ineffectiveness of psychiatric treatment had been inferred in a public policy document for fifteen years (*Action for Mental Health*, Joint Commission, 1961); and the inadequacy of community-based services was beginning to be apparent as an assumed factor in rising recidivism rates. The position of the court in Wyatt and Donaldson was taken devoid of the political reality, seemingly, as it cast the issue in simplified civil liberties terms: the State does/does not have the right to abridge the well-being of the person. Willowbrook and Dixon expanded the narrowness of the previous cases by saying that states do have responsibilities towards citizens that go beyond negating negative infringements to asserting positive systems of care.

The position of the court in these latter two cases both solves problems of individual rights and poses problems of adequacy and accountability for service provision. Since 1975, locating both an appropriate array of services and an efficient monitoring system has been problematic. For Dixon, the monitoring plan was not agreed to until 1980, assuming operation in September of that year (Mental Health Law Project Summary, July 1979–June 1981). Both accountability mechanisms and design of services were located outside the arena of state hospital determination and presumed to be adversarial rather than cooperative processes, involving continual legal negotiations over years. At stake was a question of redesign of the service delivery system, of creating and implementing after-care or alternative care services in communities where former patients had been dumped. Ironically, this very issue was central to what state governments had as their salient priority, reflecting back on the relation of the ongoing fiscal crisis to rising recidivism rates. The irony is cast in that the adversarial proceedings actually had a hidden common interest – the development of new services located in communities to offset rehospitalization for either legal or economic reasons.

During the period of heightened depopulating of state hospitals, questions were rarely raised about where patients were being sent. The legal language of the court in the 'least restrictive setting' cases simply assumed the state hospital to be the worst possible setting, but this was based more on imagery than on comparisons with other settings, most notably the private for-profit nursing home. The data from the study conducted by the Comptroller General documented a tremendous increase in the number of former psychiatric patients placed in nursing homes: between 1969 and 1974, there was a 48 per cent increase, from 607,400 to 899,500. Of the 114,200 nursing home residents under age 65, 69 per cent were diagnosed mentally disabled. Prior to 1975, nursing homes had become the largest single type of care for the discharged patient resulting in nursing homes representing a larger share of federal expenses for direct care – 29.3 per cent compared to 22.8 – than state, county and other public mental hospital costs combined (Comptroller General, 1977, p. 11).

Other systems of for-profit housing grew and developed during this same period, most notably the licensed board and care or adult home and the 'welfare hotel' or SRO (single room occupancy). Far less significant were foster care and a small smattering of half-way houses. But, for most former patients, especially those older and considered to be 'chronically disabled', community placement in fact meant involuntary relocation in a profit-run nursing home or intermediate care facility, a licensed adult home or an SRO. Often, the facilities were very large with 100–200 beds, and grossly underserviced, a view that was so widely held that the practice of community placement began to be known as reinstitutionalization. Enough scandal has been created over the years in nursing homes and adult homes to identify another critical component in mental health rhetoric covering the conversion of service delivery from institution to 'community', a criticism stated most poignantly by Charles Hynes, a Deputy Attorney General from New York:

> The discharge of mental patients from psychiatric hospitals without ensuring the delivery of aftercare services makes deinstitutionalization a procedure for patient abandonment, rather than a progressive program of patient care. (Hynes, 1977, p. 41)

Are these types of facility, organized as industries with profit as their central value, less restrictive than state hospitals? Perhaps so, but we offer as a judgment our view that imagery and rhetoric rather than systematic, comparative study of concrete daily reality was the evidential base of the lawsuits discussed above. We are not arguing in favor of state hospitals here, but rather to suggest that a political climate favoring deinstitutionalization created a rhetorical climate in which former patients were abandoned in the name of civil liberties law or compliance on the basis of some mystification about freedom from hospital confinement.

A lingering problem

In addition to failing to examine what the real options were for chronically disabled people, and presuming them to be better off outside the hospital 'no matter what', the mental health and legal reformers also overlooked another problem. Their criticism, as implied both in mental health literature surrounding the start of the community mental health centers and in litigation, focused exclusively on the service delivery system for mental health care. Note that in the transition from predominantly institution-based care to community-based care, the salient policy documents concern *where services were to be located* rather than what their essential design or operating paradigm would be (*Action for Mental Health*, Joint Commission, 1961). Put another way, psychiatrically defined services have yet to be significantly criticized as inappropriate to after-care, in part because the definition of the problem has remained medically controlled. Changing the location or setting of a psychiatrically defined set of problems from a distant hospital to a closer community-based clinic alters how those services are delivered while unintentionally validating them as appropriately construed. It also inadvertently presumes profit housing to be either benign or benevolent, paralleling management needs and the control dimensions of 'maintenance therapy.'

Challenges to medical hegemony of mental health services in after-care have been both slowly developing and indirect. Patients' needs for housing, medical care, income, legal protections and meaningful activity were subsumed under the aegis of the hospital for the duration of their stays. Virtually no provisions were made for these essential needs during the early decades of deinstitutionalization, a fact acknowledged by even the staunchest proponents of mental health ideology and confirmed by a plethora of critical studies conducted under state and federal governmental auspices. Legal investigations of the more public atrocities in nursing and adult homes, coupled with the legal decrees requiring monitoring of service provisions, indicated the paucity of protection/inspection/enforcement agencies or resources related to housing conditions for former patients, especially prior to 1975. Income provision, subsumed under SSI, but also related to Home Relief, veterans' pensions and other third party payments has been confusing and problematic for many. Health care, using Medicaid-accepting physicians, has also proven unresponsive for many former patients. The Comptroller General's report on deinstitutionalization documented the incoherence in service coordination at the federal level: the Departments of Health and Human Services, Housing and Urban Development and Labor, the Social Security Administration, Social Services, Rehabilitative Services and Medicaid/Medicare were part of the arena of practice while the community mental health centers, which were supposed to be the focal point for coordinating comprehensive systems of after-care, were often uninvolved with the deinstitutionalized population or with other service sectors (Warren *et al.*, 1974).

Similar results have been reported throughout most states – lack of adequate resources for after-care clients and unsuccessful efforts at developing state or local level coordination of the appropriate bureaucracies. In most cases, the result has been a haphazard array of residual services, crisis centers and mental health clinics whose primary function was to give and monitor medication, and emergency services provided through Social Services Departments funded under Title XX to offer protective services for adults. The legal and legislative initiatives taken in 1975 functioned in large part to call to public attention the chaotic situation that constituted a non-system of care upon community placement. Concern was shifted to development of community services that would assist former patients to remain in the community, a concern that was occasioned by economic motivation as well as humanitarian criticism of the prevailing situation. Court or legislative mandates to plan at either the organizational level or on a case by case level for discharge candidates enhanced the challenge.

The National Institute of Mental Health (NIMH) began a new program in 1977 which was a direct attempt to acknowledge the unmet needs of the chronically disabled population discharged from state hospitals. The Community Support Program (CSP) accepted as valid criticism several themes presented as reasons for existing service system deficiencies. Judith Turner and William TenHoor, NIMH central staff people responsible for CSP, identified the themes as:

1 Inadequate Definition of Service System Goals: federal leadership was required to state some positive goals for service system performance rather than allow deinstitutionalization to remain simply a process for emptying beds.
2 Fragmentation and Confusion of Responsibility: no coherent system of care existed among the many federal, state and local agencies with responsibility for service provision.
3 Lack of a Systematic Approach to Financing Community-Based Services: transfer of institutional funds to community services has not occurred, and 'Federal funding patterns . . . are a "Crazy Quilt" of conflicting jurisdictions, formulas, eligibility requirements and exclusions' (Turner and TenHoor, 1978, p. 324).
4 Lack of Commitment of 'Mainstream' Agencies to Serving the Mentally Disabled: the GAO Report documented the tendency for general service providers to presume that the mental health system would meet all needs of its former clients.

5   Lack of Effective Community Organization and Advocacy: very
    little pressure had been brought either by organized groups of
    advocates or by former patients to demand more appropriate
    services and/or access to general services (Turner and TenHoor,
    1978, pp. 322–6).

It is useful to note that the problems identified do not fault the mental
health system in terms of the appropriateness of the services which
were available, but rather turn to several other concrete problems that
are non-medical in nature. There is no clear statement about what
needs to be done in after-care, no effective or efficient means of either
delivering coordinated services or paying for them, no commitment to
providing services from locally based agencies whose resources are
needed by former patients, no organizing or advocating to press
grievances.

The response to the problems projected by NIMH was a federal
contract with nineteen state mental health agencies to create demonstration Community Support Programs whose primary target population was to be the discharged former state hospital patients. NIMH
determined that it would encourage states to develop community
support systems (CSS) through both direct contracts to provide services and to stimulate more comprehensive planning for future CSS
development. NIMH guidelines define a community support system as
'a network of caring and responsible people committed to assisting a
vulnerable population to meet their needs and develop their potentials
without being unnecessarily isolated or excluded from the community'
(quoted in Turner and TenHoor, 1978, p. 329). CSS was to become a
local system of care, with states able to improvise service delivery
models, but confined by the performance of ten essential functions
designed to ensure that the proper population is identified, an array of
needed services designed, and implementation responsibility
accounted for. Beyond the logistics, however, CSP played an important role in broadening the definition of the problem to be confronted
by applicant agencies: they went well beyond more typical medical/
psychiatric definitions of problems/solutions to identify basic needs
'for income, living arrangements, work, and socialization, assistance
in negotiating the service system' and crisis services (Turner and
TenHoor, 1978, p. 331).

By the time CSP was formulated, and the various governmental
reports critical of community-based care were issued, political consen-

sus had been reached about two implicitly vital issues: after-care services generally were under-financed and were seen as unimportant priorities by local providers, and gaps in the after-care system led to rehospitalization. Rising costs for mental health care, reflecting both growing inflation and the need to maintain old, massive physical plants, became a central economic issue related to recidivism. Inflation, fuel costs and union efforts to maintain hospital jobs were perceived, for the most part, as constant costs, as either irreducible by political decision or by lack of state control (e.g., inflation, oil costs). The climbing recidivism rates, however, together with length of stay in hospitals were more amenable to state level intervention. Psychiatric leadership, unfamiliar with the economic paradigm for decision making, and ideologically bound to a treatment regimen fixed at medical/pharmaceutical intervention (Scull, 1977, Chapter Five), began slowly to lose some of its hegemony in the field. New professionals, familiar with Office of Management and Budget or State Division of the Budget priorities, procedures and language began to occupy top level positions in state mental health departments. As the ongoing inflationary trend exacerbated the already stressed fiscal situation, cost containment became a salient theme in mental health planning and policy-making.

The thought structure of the newcomers was premised far more on systems ideology than on psychopathology, and they began to seek answers to problems of recidivism and inadequate delivery of after-care services in planning and management technology applied to service delivery models. The shift in focus, significant in terms of power and thought structures (Warren *et al.*, 1974), created an *implied* criticism of criteria used to assess 'appropriateness' of service. The concept of medical maintenance as therapeutic intervention of choice for post-discharge patients increasingly began to be seen as perhaps necessary, but certainly not sufficient. By 1978, the Commissioner of the Department of Mental Hygiene in New York acknowledged that a major assumption of psychiatrists, 'that the same high functional level achieved by patients given psychotropic drugs in the structured surroundings of the psychiatric centers could be maintained when they were released into the community', was incorrect (Prevost, 1978, p. 4). Other problems were identified: 'unable to cope with economic hardship, loneliness and lack of psychiatric, medical and social services, [many] returned to the State psychiatric centers' (Prevost, 1978, p. 506). Given substantial data by federal and state congressional researchers, the systems designers moved on to develop services constructed to maximize management values – coordination, accountability and comprehensiveness.

While these newly introduced assumed values generated a new paradigm (Kuhn, 1962) for mental health policy planning and service delivery design, they never quite replaced the old values focused on a sickness-treatment model for explaining and treating problems. Put another way, while the new approach identified problems primarily in terms of systemic deficiencies, it failed to comprehend the extent to which psychiatric orientation was entrenched in the thought structures and, therefore, the practice orientations of mental health professionals who continued to dominate the local service provider networks. As a result, there were initially no new formulations of clients' needs identified as a basis for the service delivery system designs evolved by the systems planners and managers. An ironic parallel emerged: where psychiatrically oriented programs presumed a pervasive irrationality among former patients (curbed, of course, by medication), the systems managers presumed there to be a pervasive rationality extant among service providers. Both views have proven of limited value – clients' needs in communities are far greater than psychiatric models can comprehend, just as local agency resistance and medicalized ideology far exceeds the managers' capacity (or 'trained incapacity', as Veblen termed it) to understand the local inter-organizational context as the strategic problem to be addressed in planning. For the planners/managers in central offices, the problems were clear: gaps in the system had to be identified, systems of service delivery improved, and systems of accountability put in place. To this end, C.A.O. Van Nieuwenhuijze has noted, 'Faith makes the rational system watertight' (Van Nieuwenhuijze, 1962).

The dilemma posed by the interface of local psychiatric paradigms and central office systems paradigms has been made most clear in the new community support programs, particularly in the articulation of the tasks and functions of case managers. Case management is generally accepted as the cornerstone of the new community support system approach. Even the term itself, emphasizing a manager for each client, indicates the inroads made by the new systems perspective, as does the categorical term, 'community support systems.' Case managers are supposed to perform a variety of functions, with emphasis placed on coordination of a package of services to meet clients' needs carved out on the basis of individual needs and available services. Where services are not available, or where they are not accessible to case management clients, the function to perform is identified as advocacy. This seems to make sense, until we stop to recognize that the two major providers of case management services are the out-patient clinics of state hospitals and/or local mental health agencies operating under contracts with the state. These two organizational entities are the most firmly embedded in the psychiatric paradigm. Indeed, they are also most firmly ensconced in the local interorganizational field, a fact empirically demonstrated to thwart innovation in program design or delivery (Rose, 1972; Warren *et al.*, 1974). Reluctantly, the result has been one of advocating for accessible services which are not necessarily appropriate. This occurred in order to coordinate agencies whose track records prior to CSP or CSS were known to be neglectful of former patients' community-based needs because of their perpetual reliance upon medicalized definitions of problems and their related interventions.

It is our contention that the problem of availability of services, while still existent, has been transcended by the more pervasive problem of appropriateness of services. To move forward with this phase of the struggle is to create a more supportive environment, with more fully human possibilities for former patients. To do this, it is necessary to put forward a statement about how their situation/problems are to be defined, and to orchestrate a design for services based on, and capable of being assessed by, that formulation. This book is our attempt to reformulate the field and its responsibilities. We call our approach an advocacy/empowerment design.

At first glance, it seems obvious, self-evident, that the needs of former patients would change dramatically as they left the confines of the hospital and returned to the community. For better or worse, the hospital-qua-total institution both created and met all of the patients' needs, in accordance with hospital-based definitions of reality. Certainly, in addition to what were considered mental health needs, adequate shelter and food were provided, health needs were responded to when recognized as such, and recreation and several other ancillary services also existed in most places in recent years. Of course, trade-offs existed as well – the capacity for autonomy, responsibility and self-direction was removed, particularly for those people having spent many years incarcerated in state institutions. In fact, a careful reading of the critiques of institutionalizing practices in state hospitals suggests that their overall, unintended by-product was to decontextualize the person, to contour their lives as patients in such a way as to remove or restrict their capacities for daily living in the community.

It is our belief that even the contemporary meanings attached to the term mental illness, or chronic mental illness, have this same impact. Once part of the mental hospital system, the person's capacity for self-confident assessment of real world variables becomes substantially undermined. In large part this comes about through the omnipresent insistence that the person remain on medication and continue to go to a clinic where daily life events and experiences are all too often registered by staff as responses to medication. Supplementary services in the community, from day hospital programs to vocational rehabilitation agencies, rarely acknowledge the world of poverty, inadequate housing, landlord domination, inaccessible health services, irresponsible polypharmacy, SSI decertifications and related problems that comprise the daily life of former patients. Ironically, under the rubric of reintegration into the community, many former patients have little to no contact with anyone other than people who, similar to themselves, have recently been discharged from psychiatric hospitals. Even in the newer not-for-profit community residences, program requirements regularly send people from homes to programs and back, very much like the programs for the retarded which seem designed more to alleviate community fears than to genuinely assist in habilitation.

Being transferred from a state hospital to a large community facility, often in a geographic location thoroughly unfamiliar to the ex-patient, and out of their control, does not enhance one's mental health. Rather, it builds on the already learned dependency and transfers it from state hospital workers to landlords who operate the licensed and unlicensed warehouses serving as receptacles for the state's dischargees. As business people, they share one goal in common with hospital concerns – to keep the ex-patient out of the hospital for as long as possible, under conditions which the hospital refers to as maintenance, and the owners consider management. The language of the mental health clinics and owners confirms their orientation – they refer to people as patients, and combine to treat them accordingly. Ancillary services, from case management to day programs to vocational training enterprises, most often maintain a similar outlook. The basic identity potential for the ex-patient thus emerges: she/he is encouraged and supported to stay symptom-free through medication monitoring and participation in an array of services designed to improve their functioning within the pre-existing social role of mental patient. Rather than living as a social being in a political, social, economic community, ex-patients subsist in a sub-community medicalized and static, and disguised or concealed as the community itself.

We do not believe this form of practice serves either the interests of the people for whom it was designed, nor ultimately for the mental health system itself, other than in short run gains garnered from somewhat longer stays out of the hospital in those instances where an after-care program is available. The more realistic beneficiaries are the for-profit homeowners and the service agencies, long characterized by medicalizing ideologies, who make up the local inter-organizational field of service providers. Medicalization of services supports the homeowners' commitments to manageable residents while allowing voluntary sector agencies access to state mental health dollars, thus sustaining them through budget crises created by a failing economy. Much as the voluntary sector agencies jumped to procure federal dollars in the War on Poverty, to serve a clientele for whom they had shown little to no previous interest, or relevance, the voluntary sector has joined the mental health system to provide services to former state hospital patients. And, in parallel fashion, the funding agency has continued to equate available services with appropriate services, thus maintaining the hegemony of obsolete modes of care and the service delivery models which thrive on them.

Needless to say, our approach is different. We assume that a person's behavior and emotional experiences are directly connected to biography (the person in history) and objective reality – that a person's concept of him or herself is a reflection of what they have experienced over time in particular settings combined with their current location in an objectively identifiable environment. We call what we do an advocacy/empowerment approach to practice to suggest the dialectical interaction which we presume to be constant between objective conditions and subjectivity. The use of a slash mark (/) between the two terms connotes that each is a tendency related directly to the other, that the practice comprises both, with advocacy understood to be a series of problem-focused activities arising from the lives of the people we work with that cannot be successfully negotiated through direct service provision, while empowerment is meant to characterize an ongoing process of direct interaction covering all contacts with all clients. To illustrate this briefly, the increasing practice of decertifying SSI recipients is a problem which can neither bypass the recipient nor be resolved through direct contact with the recipient – it must be taken outside the direct worker-client relationship, either to an appeal process, a fair hearing, or a courtroom. To the extent that the recipient is fully informed of what is occurring, and what the implications are for each step of advocacy that must be taken, and is authorizing each step and participating in it to his/her fullest capacity, the process of empowerment also occurs.

We chose the concept, advocacy/empowerment, to characterize our work because it reflects the practice needs of a theoretical framework which we like to think of as dialectically connecting objective conditions to historically developed forms of subjective expression (i.e., the mental patient role). We see this ongoing relation in our clients as well, expressed through their ongoing struggle focused on the coerced contradiction between patient/person. Because we see ex-patients surrounded by oppressive conditions (which will be briefly discussed below), and we see the impact of these conditions replicating the effects of incarceration on clients' self-concept and behavior, we believe that advocacy activities designed to confront the structures and ideologies of oppression are central to any direct service program – to neglect this confrontation is, in our minds, equivalent to abandoning the people. As such, we are required to identify and pursue every issue related to human and civil rights, all legal guarantees and all possible entitlements for each client, and we believe that this action must occur with the person where possible, but beyond the realm of direct practice as well; i.e., in legislative and/or legal arenas. Advocacy, thus, is issue-oriented, focused on objective conditions, and arises from the concrete daily lives of the people. It cannot be understood by itself, however, as it constitutes one major tendency within our overall framework. Advocacy attains its meaning when directly related to empowerment, since no issue can stand outside the people whose lives give rise to it, whose situations give meaning to it. Empowerment emerges as a complementary tendency to advocacy and has as its focus a process of development of the people (understood as persons in the social world, not as mental patients in community settings) which is designed to reconnect subjective responses (presentation of self, self-image, interaction patterns, etc.) to the objective conditions which form the focus for advocacy. Empowerment is perceived as a constant guide to our relationships with clients, while advocacy as a more issue-focused set of activities is a response to given conditions. In this formulation, advocacy depends upon empowerment for its substance and validity, while empowerment relies upon advocacy for its transpersonal enactment, for its substantive matter and direction.

Neither of these two dimensions to our practice has meaning without the other.

We will now move to attempt to articulate some of the derived principles of practice, based on the work of Paolo Freire. At the center of this work is the concept of struggle – of engaging in the work of transforming reality from its present configuration of oppressive, exploitative conditions to circumstances which *allow/demand* human dignity, social justice, meaningful participation of people as human beings in history. Freire's way of expressing this is to talk about the difference between people as subjects versus people as objects. In our society, where people are necessarily out of control of their relationship to survival or development – because we are out of control of the central relationship to either, or work – people are reduced to objects. Freire says that objects are known and acted upon; subjects know and act. Our work is directed towards the transformation of people turned into particular types of objects (mental patients), who are known and acted upon in particular ways, and to the transformation of the conditions which reproduce their objectification. Freire makes clear the dialectic between objective conditions/subjectivity – that changes in people cannot proceed without their engagement in changing the conditions of their oppression, hence the compatibility between his framework and our view of advocacy/empowerment.

Freire says that positive, creative work depends upon this dialectical analysis: 'The subjective aspect exists only in relation to the objective aspect (the concrete reality which is the object of analysis). Subjectivity and objectivity thus join in a dialectical unity producing knowledge in solidarity with action and vice versa' (1968, p. 22). Consciousness, or growing knowledge of the unity, is based upon growing solidarity of the people as subjects. Freire cautions against sectarianism of the right and left. The right bases the possibilities of the future on the 'facts' of the past seen uncritically (the ultimate rehabilitation program for mental patients), while the sectarian left ignores the experience of the people in declaring the future to be presently in effect: 'Both types of sectarian, treating history in an equally proprietary fashion, end up without the people – which is another way of being against them' (1968, p. 23).

In opposition to closed 'circles of certainty' or undebatable perspectives, positive practice requires dialogue, an entering into the reality of lived and perceived experiences of the people. Entering this reality, however, does not occur in a vacuum – it begins with a critical consciousness of objective conditions and their impact on peoples' lives, patterns of behavior and self-concept. We begin with these understandings of state hospitals, social control, the medical model, mental patienthood and profit housing as objective facts of oppression and proceed from there. Our challenge is to invite people to join in their own/our struggle, a task that requires us to understand the stakes/benefits/costs involved for the person acting out mental patienthood as a survival strategy, as a way of life. We must understand submergence in a socially constructed oppressive role. To do this we must examine our own lives first (man/woman, parent/child, husband/ wife) as an avenue for comprehending what submergence means, and what its incentives and costs are. From within our own situation, we must reflect on Freire's comment: 'In order for the oppressed to be able to wage the struggle for their liberation, they must perceive the reality of oppression, not as a closed-world from which there is no exit, but as a limiting situation which they can transform'. (1968, p. 34.)

With ourselves as well as with the participants in our Project, we must devise ways of creating a multitude of lower level 'limit situations' rather than focus on the whole social structure as the only target of change. Put another way, as we pointed out above, we must redefine problems consistent with real needs. Yet we must do this based upon our capacity to comprehend their situation: how do we find ways to develop opportunities for the experience of human dignity? For the opportunity to engage in human (as opposed to mental patient) activity? It is clear that humanizing activity relates their experience as objects to the objective world through a dignifying process which we describe as empowerment. All activities and interactions must presume this central premise – that our participants are oppressed persons who, through their historical experience, have largely incorporated or internalized the content and process of their oppression as part of their identities (= submergence). Submergence is the internalization of a view of reality which contradicts peoples' interests/needs. According to Freire, 'Submerged in reality, the oppressed cannot perceive clearly the "order" which serves the interests of the oppressors whose image they have internalized.' (1968, p. 48.) Similarly, 'Self-depreciation is another characteristic of the oppressed, which derives from their internalization of the opinion the oppressors hold of them.' (1968, p. 49.)

Our task is to build enough support for people to allow them to allow us to see how they perceive the world. This is a prerequisite step for an empowering process. In our program, we try to do this through raising issues and questions about concrete, real life issues; through participation in socially useful activity; through dialogue in groups and community meetings. Issues raised from the empowerment process to advocacy levels must simultaneously be returned to their origin through activity which embodies both tendencies. Case management, following similar principles, continues to create limited situations related to daily life, usually focused on legal rights and entitlements. In each situation, the challenge is to find the vehicle for transmitting information, supporting the struggle of the person to grasp the material in relation to their reality and to encourage movement from a status of being known/acted upon to an experience of knowing/acting.

As we indicated in the beginning, it is necessary to have a clearly articulated conceptual framework to create a practice directed towards meeting the needs identified above. The first section of this book is our effort to communicate that framework to you. It is composed of three related chapters: the first of these presents an alternative perception and definition of the problems to be addressed or an alternative perspective on reality; the second chapter identifies a set of practice principles which derive from.the problem definition or statement of needs adopted in the first chapter; and the third chapter discusses the integration of the needs statement and practice principles as a social action strategy.

Section II presents five different arenas in which advocacy/empowerment practice can be implemented in the field of mental health after-care. The first two practice chapters, on case management and day programs, identify the two most common programs of after-care. The case management chapter focuses primarily on working with individuals, elaborating the theoretical material where appropriate. The day program chapter focuses on working with groups and furthers the theory specifically in that direction. Both the case management and day program chapters confront typical programs which exist in most communities where former patients have been dispatched. While our practice concerns correspond in form to these typical patterns of service delivery, in content and in daily process, we believe that our approach to problem definition and practice is significantly different and constitutes an entirely contradictory paradigm from that employed by most mental health after-care programs.

Following the two direct practice chapters there are three other practice chapters, all generally included under the 'indirect practice' rubric. These three chapters focus more on the advocacy dimension of the advocacy/empowerment approach to practice, but obviously are not isolated from the daily lives of former patients and direct practice workers. These chapters, on legal advocacy and organizing, program evaluation, and community organization, focus on the more overtly political dimensions of daily life and confront the need for political activity in each area targeted for special attention.

We conclude with a brief summary based on inter-organizational theory which we see as necessary to organizational survival. It sets forth the framework for construction of inter-organizational strategy development for advocacy/empowerment-oriented people and programs. This framework is premised on a conflict perspective which we see as necessary for alternative agencies to embrace in order to avoid either cooptation or a premature demise. We hope to suggest pathways for advocacy/empowerment program or agency survival since the struggle for progressive development is one continually in need of support in the face of certain threats from conventional provider systems.

Section I

The Theory of Advocacy/ Empowerment Practice

CHAPTER 1

Problem Definition – A Theory and Orientation

Essential to the development of a positive practice in mental health after-care is a precise formulation of clients' needs or a problem definition. Clarity about a statement of needs provides added information about anticipated obstacles to meeting those needs, both at the client and systemic levels. To accomplish this preliminary task, it becomes necessary to create what we refer to as a 'problem definitional' level of theory. Problem defining theory mediates between the more global theory of society which establishes a larger context for understanding the broad policy issues and direct implications (for an elaboration of this approach, see Vicente Navarro, 'Health and the Corporate Society', *Social Policy*, Jan/Feb, 1975), and the articulation of practice theory, the task of the next chapter of this book.

Problem definitional theory is a prerequisite to practice as it establishes both a direction and a baseline for evaluation of practice activities. At a programmatic level, it is necessary to recognize that all providers of services operate out of one or another approach to defining clients' needs (i.e., problems) as well as a structure for delivering services. Properly construed, a service agency or organization is simultaneously a social system of interlocking roles and functions and the embodiment of an ideology or identifiable thought structure that frames the way the organization perceives social reality. These often underlying assumptions contour agencies' perceptions of clients' existence, and establish the parameters of the functions they have to perform vis-à-vis one another (Warren *et al.*, 1974; Rose, 1972). The thought structure of an agency, while most often implicit or concealed, contains the problem (needs) definition or theoretical formulation that underlies all services and client-worker interactions.

The thought structure also provides the formal and implied rationality for the infrastructure of the organization and for its location within the inter-organizational network at the community level. As Warren and his co-authors state, the institutionalized thought structure constitutes, 'a common frame of reference regarding the nature of social reality, of American society, of social problems, and of efforts at social change and human betterment' (Warren *et al.*, 1974, p. 19).

The thought structure or set of operating assumptions which typically characterize the commonly found health and social service agencies in most American communities is widespread: its hidden, but practised beliefs assert the basic soundness and equity of American society, its institutions, and patterns of behavior. The concealed social validation for our political economy and social structure is found in the overwhelming commonality in the way agencies define the needs/problems of their clients. In the Warren *et al.* study of fifty-four agencies in nine cities, people either needing service or failing to fit into already established service delivery patterns were defined as defective; their difficulties in living, rather than resulting from poverty, underemployment, discrimination or inadequate care were seen as results of their individual behaviors or values. These were either defined or, more likely, assumed to be causal. Whether the defect was located in individuals' intellect, personality, discipline or values or in family structure or neighborhood, one or more of these factors were taken to be the determinants of the client's social position in society. Agency responses, in the form of programs and service designs, for example, were incapable of recognizing poverty as an inherent structural characteristic of our society; incapable of recognizing race, sex, age or handicap as structurally and historically determined aspects or characteristics of American society. Problem definitional assumptions, validating inequity and/or discrimination, found their expression in paradigms of practice which carried with them practice technologies and assessment methods that turned out to be self-serving. They were incapable of critical reflection beyond the agency parameters of perceived-defined clients' defects. Rose's earlier research on the Community Action Program identified the same phenomenon: in this case, agencies directed by federal mandate to engage in social change-defined services instead delivered their common litany of residual services based on individual defect conceptual models (Rose, 1972).

The scope of commonality in problem definition across different types of agencies, operating in different service domains, in different cities was so typical that Warren *et al.*, referred to the pattern as an 'institutionalized thought structure' (Warren *et al.*, 1974, p. 19). While agencies as different in their areas of special interest as the public schools, the urban renewal agency, the anti-poverty program, the major mental health planning agency and the health and welfare council were present in most communities, and had allocated various functions and tasks among them that differed widely, their locus of common understanding was in their operational paradigms of practice, all founded upon a set of basic assumptions invalidating their clients and validating the social system (Warren *et al.*, 1974).

Upon closer examination, these agencies appeared to have established 'legitimate' domains of domination locally, dividing the turf according to functions and prerogatives, claimed expertise and professional leadership. What was found to exist was an informal, yet pooled hegemony over community activity and decision making related to service design and delivery, a rather loosely orchestrated collaboration determined to protect individual agency turf from infringement or criticism.

Agreement among service providers at the level of basic assumptions about clients, and ultimate responsibility for problems, allows agencies to attribute program failure either to client defects ('Blaming the Victim', as it has become known – see Ryan, 1976) or to a form of quantitative or administrative/management rationality. This latter dimension manifests itself in continuous demands for more funds, more staff, more local control over program decisions, etc. Funding agencies, from the vertical or extra-community system (Warren, 1963, Chapter 8) at the state or federal levels, most often share the institutionalized thought structure. In the unfolding of federal and/or state programs, vertical input rarely relates to problem definitions, especially so long as funding is available. During those periods, the nature of criticism, such as it was, assumed the problems that existed were related to lack of adequate coordination, insufficient comprehensiveness, and/or inappropriate representation on advisory boards, all examples of what we have referred to as administrative or management rationality. As fiscal constraint gradually increases, the demand for more effective coordination is joined by a growing interest in greater program monitoring and in improving accountability mechanisms. This introduces some tension between vertical system funding agencies and horizontal or local system providers of services.

As fiscal crisis continues unabated, however, the vertical system

becomes more determined to locate measures of program effectiveness tied to cost containment. As we noted in the Introduction, this
trend has accelerated in public mental health care. Its pronounced
manifestation is reflected in the increase of people whose training is in
disciplines and/or professions outside the typical mental health–social
service preparatory schools. As a result, incoming policy planners,
program developers and managers and decision makers have little
specific commitment to the existing particular forms of individual
defect explanatory paradigms that comprise the prevailing institutionalized thought structure. Corresponding to basic values espoused
by State Bureaus of the Budget, or the Office of Management and
Budget at the federal level, their focus has been on management by
objectives, fiscal accountability mechanisms, cost containment and
system development.

The 'New Breed' of mental health policy-makers, however, are not
consciously predisposed against prevailing individual defect models,
since their systems training and management outlook contains no
ideological or substantive critique of the structure of society. Instead,
their professional set of responsibilities initially leads them to accept
the institutionalized thought structure of the local provider systems
and then, later on, to begin to question it on the basis of cost-
effectiveness measures of program outcomes. As noted above, recidivism rates probably stand as the most critical evidence available, with
lesser variables including average length of stay on inpatient services,
length of time between hospitalizations, altering discharge planning to
avoid nursing home placements, etc.

Because all socially legitimated professional training accepts prevailing ideology uncritically (Berger and Luckmann, 1967), and extends it by posing the functions of the professions as technical problem
solving (Marcuse, 1964; O'Connor, 1973), the 'New Breed' simultaneously struggles to improve services that are cost-efficient while
having no substantively new criteria for determining what services will
either be of value to clients or cost-efficient. This phenomenon of
increasingly technical management systems without precise theoretical focus creates the opening for our problem definitional level of
theory, a conceptual articulation of needs that offers a new paradigm
for service design, implications for practice and bases for evaluation
and training. Its non-medical, non-institutional orientation provides
cost-effectiveness rationality to complement its programmatic logic.
By the accident of definition of the problem, it begins with a potential

quantitative (cost-effective) advantage; it has no salaries for medically trained psychiatric staff.

Basic statement of needs

A large number of studies have been done over the years which describe the process of becoming a mental patient in a state psychiatric hospital. Perhaps the most detailed account, *Asylums*, by Erving Goffman (1961), demonstrated the connection between defining a problem in a particular fashion – in this case, seeing dysfunctional behavior as a medical entity – and fashioning an entire social system whose ultimate function is to confirm that definition and rule out all possible alternatives (see Berger and Luckmann, 1967, on 'nihilation'). An absolute prerequisite to the smooth operation of any total institution is the process through which its incarcerated participants learn the conceptual and behavioral parameters of the new social reality they must accept in order to survive.

In the mental hospital, the patients must come to accept their situation or 'problem' as mental illness, as a disease which they had somehow acquired which, from that point forward, dictates the realm of possibilities for them, as interpreted by hospital staff. Staff, in turn, must produce mental patients out of troubled people in order for their own professional identities to make sense. Once the activity of production of the mental patient has occurred, thus validating staff and reciprocally invalidating patients (by turning them into adaptive, objectified response units), the drama of ongoing social interaction simply reproduces the inequality, domination and manipulation inherently built into practice premised on the medical-psychiatric model.

At the center of the process of becoming a mental patient is what we call 'decontextualization', the severing of the patient's subjectivity from the objective historical context that frames and contours human social life. Another way of looking at decontextualization is to see it as removal from social historical reality. The reduction to isolated, asocial existence is bounded not by history, but by a belief system committed to psychopathology, medical hegemony and somatic interventions such as shock treatment, drugs and pseudo-medical examinations. Decontextualized experiences of daily life also become saturated with new language, the language of mental illness, which contains such concepts as symptoms, regression, decompensation, acting out, etc. These are all terms used to reduce social reality to intrapsychic distortion. In place of living one's life, however painfully, one now 'functions' more or less well, and according to a set of rules and standards which have no bearing on genuine rehabilitation or return to social-community living, but rather reflect management priorities decided by staff to be in patients' best interests.

When examined closely, the behaviors necessary to becoming a good patient, especially years ago, are behaviors exactly opposite to those needed by a person to survive in the social world of community life. The good patient is docile, acquiescent and adaptive to commands both overt and subtle. He/she is overwhelmingly dependent upon staff, socially naive regarding rights and/or entitlements and demoralized or frightened to be him/herself. After a time, the externally imposed new social order becomes incorporated subjectively – the problem definition coercively held out is tacitly accepted. But in the process, the patient undergoes an experience of anomie – of an abrupt withdrawal of norms and forms (universe of meaning) that communicated the exigencies of daily social life as he/she knew it before entering the hospital. The experience of such extraction of one's known universe of meaning is profound. Even conventional common sense communicates this to us when any significant threat of social change is raised in the common assumption that any departure from the routine represents absolute chaos. Rather than chaos, however, the hospital institutes systematic order, and the patient's experience of heightened anomie together with the hospital's rigid definition of reality combine to produce the mental patient. Any conscious or non-conscious effort at resistance, whether expressed behaviorally, emotionally or conceptually is understood to be part of the patient's symptom pattern, and thus brings about increased treatment responses designed to attain manageability or control.

So as one gains the knowledge and skills necessary to survive in and adapt to the world of the hospital, one loses those same capabilities for life in the community. Seeing oneself as sick, having lost the ability to link subjective experience to objective circumstances (decontextualization), and seeing the necessity to perceive quickly the expectations of power holders, the mental patient's potential for independent or interdependent social life in the community is thoroughly compromised. Their social being, or personhood, is overwhelmed by their patienthood; their active participation in and consciousness of historical/social reality is overwhelmed by their passive acquiescence or functional adaptation to and acknowledgment of their own invalid state. They have been disconnected from ongoing social existence, almost as if their capacity to engage in the process of struggling to live meaningfully has been surgically severed. It is exactly this objective aspect of utter oppression, *behaviorally and conceptually*, that constitutes what is called 'chronic disability', or what we prefer to call 'institutionalization'. In our view, it is a prerequisite to understanding practice to comprehend the experience to which people have been subjected, and to see their histories in the hospitals as a central ingredient in designing practice activities with them.

The other aspect of daily life that converges to form the matrix of understanding how to define the problem properly is much easier to elaborate. It requires that we remember that mental patients, before entering the hospital, during their stay and after their release, are essentially like us – human and therefore social historical beings. In this capacity, so estranged from them because of their hospitalization, they have needs/interests exactly as we do. Simply put, those needs include: adequate income; adequate, safe, supportive housing; nutritious food; adequate clothing; varying knowledge of their rights and entitlements to benefits and programs; legal protection; and the choice to participate in socially meaningful interaction with others who treat them with dignity and respect. We want to stress that ex-patients need those resources socially, as persons living in the community, and not psychiatrically, as patients, temporarily residing outside the hospital. As such, any effort to deliver social resources in a psychiatric manner constitutes a situation in which the peoples' needs may be met, but in a way which contradicts their interests (e.g., acquiring a Medicaid card for psychiatric clinic visits only).

At this point, a slight departure is necessary to further articulate the difference between needs and interests as these terms were used in the preceding paragraph. Statements of need are common enough among mental health and social agencies. What such statements rarely take into account is that the way in which they define needs and/or construct services is entirely confined by their institutional thought structures. Where those thought systems are premised on some assumption of the inherent defectiveness of their patients or clients, then the orientation towards defining needs will be confined within the descriptive parameters of their thought structure. In practice, this is commonly reflected in mental health providers' coupling psychiatric focus to community resources, or psychiatric determination of generic needs such as those outlined above. Sheltered housing has as its basis not some form of care for those unable to live independently, but rather the assurance that psychotropic medical regimens will be followed. Case management, rather than being built on advocacy and/or empowerment principles designed to guarantee the essential dignity and benefits needed, instead focuses on ensuring ongoing linkage to mental health clinics and other treatment outlets. These psychiatrically-oriented services, based on continued attribution of, and reinforcement for, mental patienthood as an enduring identity, act against the interests of the former patient. They continue the pattern of enslaved dependence/hegemony; they disregard the exploitation inevitably built-in to profit housing arrangements; and they support passive dependence upon staff where it is not needed, thus manipulating the former patient into continued subservience.

The interests of former patients are quite different. Former patients require the social resources described above to be delivered in a way which recognizes their hospital experiences as oppressive and debilitating, and which works with them to regain their human vitality and active participation in locating what they require. The interests of the ex-patient are, therefore, complex in nature, reflecting the experience/existence of the ex-patient understood as a human being, not as a manufactured commodity/mental patient. The use of the term 'complex' here is intended: interests are interpreted in a way which recognizes the ex-patients' status as members of a class. The concept of needs depicted here is infused with the necessity to begin with material conditions – housing, food, health care, meaningful social relations and activity – as a basis for understanding subjective responses. We are saying, more simply, that the ex-patient, like us, cannot be understood apart from his/her context, and that the form of self-expression used in any context is a crystallization of the social relations contained therein. One's identity, therefore, emerges as a critical commentary on a social network rather than standing as a statement about an autonomous individual.

What we mean here is that the behaviour of the 'chronic' ex-patient must be seen in two ways at the same time. It must be understood as a learned survival strategy, as historical baggage that the person brings with him/her from the hospital; and it must be seen as a result of the social relations she/he is and has been involved in over time. This dimension can be elaborated by seeing in the typical behavior patterns of the ex-patient the reciprocal functioning of the typical behaviour patterns of the mental health professional; one cannot be understood apart from the other. When we examine the ideological and organizational bases from and in which typical mental health theory and practice emerge, we can see the larger context of social control, oppression and domination of both workers, confined to medical model paradigms, and their products – the institutionalized or chronic ex-patients. Because the ideology and organizational environments are similar across states (see David Rosenhan's fine work, 'On Being Sane in Insane Places,' 1973), the conditions of life for former patients discharged into communities across the country are quite similar. The ex-patients, then, while existing as individuals, simultaneously are essential members of a class.

Because we think this issue is both complex and vital, it will be explained here at greater length. This will be done by drawing a distinction between what we refer to as essential aspects of former patients' lives and pragmatic dimensions. Following the theoretical distinctions drawn above, the essential components or tendencies in ex-patients' lives are the political and economic conditions which all endure in common that aggregate them as members of a common class. In addition to the common base of long term hospitalization and its impact on self-confidence and self-image, and its effect on how reality is perceived (i.e., internalization of the medical model), there are common social conditions: placement in profit-organized long term care facilities of one kind or another (varying by degree of regulation); dependency on third party payments for medical care; dependency upon continued eligibility and recertification for SSI or other forms of public assistance; and, most likely, continuation on psychotropic drugs. In this complex organization-infused and dominated existence, ex-patients are subjugated, exploited and manipulated in common, as members of a class, and the contours of their daily lives are conditioned by these oppressive, coerced factors. Because this is so, and uniform, we refer to this dimension as political – it contains the objective parameters for subjective expression.

In the assumption that objective, historical conditions contour the parameters of everyday life, and establish the bases for individual subjective experience and expression, we create a bond between ex-patients, even the severely disabled, and ourselves. The bond is forged by acknowledging the essential human quality that comes from being part of history, from being socially alive, and therefore actually or potentially a creative participant in shaping the future, even in a microcosmic context. It is in this socially human crucible that the enduring, inherent and inextricable bond is made between political life and personal or pragmatic life. In our perspective, each of these aspects of every person is woven into the other, each a tendency without the capacity to lose its omnipresent life. While both are present, however, they are not equally active participants in shaping daily experience. Quite obviously, the historical/political or objective dimension – bringing with it an ongoing political economy, culture, ideology and social role structure – plays a pre-eminent role in determining the personal exigencies experienced by all of us. Particular patterns of self-expression, such as the docile, acquiescing behaviors common to mental patient identity, reflect the particular forces which dominate existence; self expression and personal experience, therefore, emerge as a social relational/political statement about each of us.

Where the patterns of subjective experience and self-expression fully inculcate the political environment in its objectified forms, our behavior functions to reproduce that environment and our place within it (mental patient, husband, wife, parent/child, for example). Where our form of self-expression is in conflict with the exigencies of the political environment, we pose a challenge or threat to it. Such a position requires some form of response from those political contexts invested in domination and control.

The unwritten rule is that people must both behave appropriately or according to the dictates of the social role structures of such a society, and they must perceive reality in such a way that the behaviors they embody appear natural or normal. Peter Berger and Thomas Luckmann describe societal response to abandonment of this latter ideological element, which they call a 'conceptual machinery,' similar in the individual to what we have earlier described in organizations as an 'institutional thought structure':

Therapy entails the application of conceptual machinery to ensure that actual or potential deviants stay within the institutionalized definitions of reality, or, in other words, to prevent the 'inhabitants' of a given universe from 'emigrating.' It does this by applying the legitimating apparatus to individual 'cases'. . . . What interests us here, however, is the conceptual aspect of therapy. Since therapy must concern itself with deviations from the 'official' definitions of reality, it must develop a conceptual machinery to account for such deviations and to maintain the realities thus challenged. This requires a body of knowledge that includes a theory of deviance, a diagnostic apparatus, and a conceptual system for the 'cure of souls.' (Berger and Luckmann, 1967, pp. 112–13)

Sharing in the common universe of meaning, as the background for our own socialization, creates the basis for shared action. The particular experience of the ex-patient, in the process of becoming a 'mental patient', is an example of the political role of therapeutic enterprise in personal life.

Institutionalization, combining coercive physical relocation and rearrangement of thought to comply with a dictated reality, extends the therapeutic mode of social control. Berger and Luckmann address this form of internal domination:

Such a conceptual machinery (therapy) permits its therapeutic application by the appropriate specialists and may also be internalized by the individual afflicted with the deviant condition. Internalization itself will have therapeutic efficacy . . . . Successful therapy establishes a symmetry between the conceptual machinery and its subjective appropriation in the individual's consciousness; it resocializes the deviant into the objective reality. (1967, p. 114)

The behavior patterns of the institutionalized ex-patients reflect their resocialization into acceptable patterns of thought and action. Severed from the knowledge of the objective conditions of reality, and medicated beyond its emotional impact, the ex-patient unwillingly serves the state by assisting to decrease state budgets; by serving as the conduit for transferring public funds to the private profit sector; and by being the 'beneficiary' of federal-state funding programs (SSI, Medicaid) which transfer power to the federal level.

These characteristics, coupled with the more commonly acknowledged matters of material need and program responses in the forms of profit housing and therapeutic activities, become the objective universe that extends the worst aspects of hospital life into the community. The pervasive influence of these objective factors reinforces the demoralized self, expressed pragmatically by the ex-patient. It is exactly this demoralized self, communicated as mental patient identity/self-expression, that becomes the focus of treatment by most after-care provider systems. In the implementation of programs which, either overtly or subtly, are founded upon a medical/

therapeutic definition of reality, providers reinforce the decontextualization of hospital life. Taking the mental patient to be the same as
the person disassociates mental health and other social service workers
from their responsibility for their own activity. Accountable to both a
profession and to an agency which employs people socialized into
professional roles and thought structures, the workers become as
disconnected from their real activities – consciously understood and
chosen – as are their products, the ex-patients. Where the absolute
confrontation with the material or objective circumstances of daily life
is not seen as the basis for subjective expression, the essential political
and the pragmatic components of living are transposed. In this process
of turning reality on its head, the expressions of self of the ex-patients
are presumed to be the determinants of their objective situation. The
'treatment' strategy accompanying this outlook thus asserts that the
subjectivity of the ex-patient, as manifests in their self-expression,
becomes the target for intervention. Therapy, drugs and all rehabilitation programs are premised on this peculiar, but all too understandable, belief. Their effort is directed to reshaping the subjectivity of
former patients by improving their behavioral functioning *within* their
existing social roles, thus reaffirming the very aspects of the person
they find most abhorrent, and reproducing the most offensive aspects
of the environment.

Alternative practice

Our alternative position follows another road entirely. It asserts the
primacy of reconnection to objective circumstances as the central
problem to be addressed, as an ever-present theme to be interwoven in
every aspect of practice. Rather than conceal its nature in subjectivism, it demands that ex-patients be understood as social, historical
beings. Validation, a central value of this position, derives its meaning
from the concept of reconnection. People, not mental patients, exist in
history as actual or potential producers or participants in their own
lives. Validation is communicated through the processes of reconnecting people to their sociality, disconnecting them from their objectified
or reified status as mental patients. Pragmatic or existential differences, while not denied, are relegated to secondary importance, as
commonalities, based on class position, rise to the position of primacy,
and the essential aspects of daily life that bond people together become

the data base for creating support networks among people.

The task of engaging people as producer/participants in comprehending and acting on their contextual environment differs dramatically from working to improve an individual patient's functioning, even though both may claim to improve the quality of life and self-image of the former patient. One way to view the scope and depth of the difference is to examine the meaning of being a producer-participant as compared to being a service consumer-attender. The producer-participant, which embodies our design, must come to know the active ingredients which compose her/his social world of immediate influence. The framework for development of such a view is open-ended, confined by limits in *our* practice and by the interaction of resources available and decisions to act. It implies a conscious strategy for action, not an acquiescence to dictates.

It is important to see that we are neither moving towards some predetermined model of what a proper adult or proper ex-mental patient might be, and thus subjecting people to manipulation, nor are we posing some rhetorical infinity such as 'the liberated person.' In contrast, we submit that each of us can come to increase our knowledge of our historical and immediate context, and with active support, stategically placed into it as participants-producers of what the outcome might be. We are not claiming that a group of ex-mental patients can transform poverty: we are suggesting that knowing that poverty has much to do with their present situation can produce different concrete and/or social relational outcomes than seeing their condition as the result of an incurable mental disease.

More conventionally, service providers would like their clientele to become more adroit consumers of services. Consuming mental health or social services, however adeptly, communicates an entirely different outcome than engagement in a process of participation as a producer. There is a striking parallel between consumers of services and consumers of commodities: both are out of control of what they consume; both stand outside the determinants of the process of production; both act in response to a definition of their needs outside their conscious control; and both are passive recipients of the interaction which reproduces existing power relations. Navarro describes the effect of consumption on identity in the following way: consumption, whether of goods or services, is the residue allocated to workers and non-workers by capitalist production, from which the workers are removed as a source of power and control. Being coerced into consumption creates feelings of helplessness, malaise and pessimism (Navarro, 1983, p. 114). Consuming services is a process through which the consumer must take on the problem definition of the provider, much like the situation described above in relation to inpatient care. What we want to stress here is that the process of consuming the service consumes the person: the likelihood of the consumer transcending or transforming the given universe of meaning established by the provider is very little, indeed. Marcuse captures this activity of service provision and consumption in a manner which aptly describes the mental health clinic-former patient relationship:

> To the degree to which they correspond to the given reality, thought and behavior express a false consciousness, responding to and contributing to the preservation of a false order of facts. (Marcuse, 1964, p. 145)

Marcuse's concern is with the diminishing capacity to develop critical analyses of society and its impact on peoples' thought and behavior, a concern which we share and which we think can be applied to mental health after-care.

In programs where people have been reduced to mental patients, where presentation of self or, in our case here, mental patient identity and the essence of a person are presumed to be the same, both the person involved and the workers become one-dimensional or flattened out. There is little to no room for creativity, for development, for change. The world of the possible becomes reduced to the situation at hand: stasis, paralysis, and demoralization occur. In a program which medicalizes poverty, exploitation, domination and abuse, the contrast and potential contradiction between the given and the possible is collapsed or crushed. When the range of needs is defined in terms of medicalized interests, those needs which can be satisfied by this model are merged with those which cannot, creating a false universe of satisfaction (Marcuse, 1964) or a defective or resistant patient. In this typical pattern, the concepts of patients and needs are 'reduced' according to Marcuse and these reduced concepts come to govern the analysis of human reality. The result is that these ideas convey

> a false consciousness – a concreteness isolated from the conditions which constitute its reality. In this context, the operational treatment of the concept assumes a political function. The individual and his [sic] behavior are analyzed in a therapeutic sense – adjustment to his [sic] society. Thought and expression, theory and practice are to be brought in line with the facts of

his [sic] existence without leaving room for the conceptual critique of these facts. (Marcuse, 1964, p. 107)

Consuming mental health after-care services, free from a conceptual critique of the objective reality of hospitalization and of post-hospital conditions, is to consume a false reality made up of false facts. Living that false reality reaffirms the mental patient role, the mental health worker role, and the set of institutions and ideology which created both of them. When we ask the question – who benefits? – we can see that the primary recipients are outside the equation. They include the profit accumulated by landlords and pharmaceutical industries; the savings sustained by state governments; and the comforts extended to the professional hierarchies dominated by psychiatry.

What, then, is to be done? What we are postulating as necessary is a practice paradigm which incorporates the larger contextual analysis presented in the Introduction with the problem definition established here. This approach to practice must combine some a priori understanding of former patients' hospitalization experience with a clear formulation of their needs – real, material needs – as residents of a community. It must seek to accept what former patients communicate about their lives as statements of self-expression *and* their internalized view of the perception of them held by powerful others in their past and present environments. And it must devise ways of reflecting this shared communication back to the former patients in a critical manner, so that the interaction neither reinforces the oppressive reality nor reproduces it. To formulate such a practice requires a theory of practice consonant with the broader theory and problem definitional theory presented above. For this purpose, we turn now to our orientation toward practice based on the work of Paolo Freire (Freire, 1968).

CHAPTER 2

Practice Theory – Bridging the Gap to Action

The task of this practice theory chapter will be to articulate a set of principles which formulate the creative bases for working with ex-patients. From our perspective, the principles we discuss here have far greater application and can be generalized to other populations parti-cipating in direct services.

The responsibilities we have include developing a framework for practice which validates the person, reconnects her/him to the *objective context* in which she/he lives, legitimates the impact of psychiatric history or self-expression, and engages the person in a process of transformation. The transforming process must confront the elements or ingredients existing in the present context which maintain or reproduce mental patient functioning/thwart personal development. The process aims to support an increasing autonomy and capacity for interdependence and act against isolation; to support collectivity or network building and to deny the primacy of individual functional performances. At the same time, the principles must not romanticize the ex-patient, must not deny the impact of hospitalization by assum-ing the person is free and automatically capable of full autonomous living – unless the person demands this perception and refuses to participate in available services. In the pursuit of a set of internally related practice principles which embody the values espoused here, we came upon the work of Paolo Freire.

Freire is an educator. His early work was devoted to literacy training of both urban and rural poor people in his native country, Brazil. Because we feel that all social interactions, and particularly those types of interaction which are purposive, are teaching/learning exchanges, we find Freire's work of inestimable value to us. His theoretical framework, his basis for intervention, is dialectical: objective historical conditions are seen as central to subjective expressive experience, each posited as a relation of the other.

In the introduction to Freire's *Pedagogy of the Oppressed*, Richard Shaull says, Freire

> came to realize that their [the poor] ignorance and lethargy were the direct product of the whole situation of economic, social and political domination – and of the paternalism – of which they were victims . . . they were kept 'submerged' in a situation in which [such] critical awareness and response were practically impossible. (in Freire, 1968, pp. 10–11)

There are distinct parallels between the submerged and oppressive existence of Brazilian poor and of former psychiatric patients: the objective conditions of poverty and exploitation have already been described, as have the repercussions of internalization of the medical model. Interactions between ex-patients and landlords or ex-patients and most service providers constitute tutoring sessions in which the people either reaffirm their knowledge of their own disabilities and frailty or begin to affirm their social historical being, their right to participate in living as conscious active persons.

If we look at this in a more simply stated manner, we can say that all social exchange has a political content: whether conscious or not, it expresses a commitment to or a critique of a social order (Gouldner, 1970). Shaull puts it this way:

> There is no such thing as a neutral educational process. Education either functions as an instrument which is used to facilitate the integration of the younger generation into the logic of the present system and bring about conformity to it, or it becomes 'the practice of freedom', the means by which men and women deal critically and creatively with reality and discover how to participate in the transformation of their world. (in Freire, 1968, p. 15)

Quite obviously, we think the process of working with ex-patients contains these same diametrically opposed possibilities. As we have indicated above, we believe the typical services provided, whether from the medical or more recent psychosocial models, reproduce the behavior/thought patterns (social roles) inculcated in people as part of their hospitalization. In trying to reduce unmanageable or disagreeable behaviour, thought or mood to intrapsychic distortion alone, or in trying to improve the behavioural functioning of a manageable commodity or a contained identity (i.e., the mental patient), these two approaches attempt to integrate and sustain former patients in an environment characterized by domination, exploitation and manipulation – and to keep them 'submerged' in the belief that such an environment is either benign and/or irrelevant to their human experience.

Freire claims that people are characterized by an '*ontological vocation*', an unending struggle of oppressed people 'for freedom and justice, and . . . to recover their lost humanity' (in Freire, 1968, p. 28). In this formulation, dehumanization, or the negation of the people as manifest in injustice, poverty, exploitation and domination is understood as concrete historical fact rather than as an inevitability. Historical fact is socially created and thus is capable of being known and changed by people. Freire encompassed a notion of the political dimension of personal experience – he says that oppressed people have an interest in transforming their world; that their interest is inherently part of their humanity; and that it seeks a direction premised on justice and freedom. These qualities are inescapably social in that they exist in people socially (and cannot be individually owned) and are expressed in history. They also emerge as responses to oppressive conditions which, Freire says, are a distortion of human development, a perversion of our 'Ontological Vocation.' The task is to uncover this perversion objectively, to reflect critically on its existence and the causes of its existence, and to join together to transform the conditions which produce, maintain and reproduce the situation together with the mystifications (submergence) which sustain it.

Of paramount importance is the necessity to trust the people to follow their perception of a reality which will produce the freedom they seek, and yet to comprehend that their perception may be overwhelmingly distorted by the conditions which shape their lives. These conditions include the concretely real circumstances of poverty and domination, together with the submergence that rationalizes their subjugation as 'natural' or deserved because of their 'mental illness' or 'chronic disability'. Freire expresses this point:

> this does not necessarily mean that the oppressed are unaware that they are downtrodden. But their perception of themselves as oppressed is impaired by their submersion in the reality of oppression. (in Freire, 1968, p. 30)

Mental patients and ex-patients share in common the characteristics of an *object: they are known and acted upon*. Freire contrasts 'objects' with 'subjects': Subjects know and act. Responsible subjects continue to know their social world and act to transform it while accountable objects consume aspects of their social world and exist to reproduce it. Objects – whether ex-patients or the workers whose identities require that former patients remain that way – are commodities, things manufactured to maintain and reproduce social reality in its present form. Subjects, in contrast, are dynamic; subjects are participants, creators, producers. Practice, or *praxis* as Freire calls it, involves *the transformation of objects into subjects*, of consumers into producers. It applies simultaneously to workers and client populations.

Transformation is an unending process. It has no predetermined or non-emergent goal, nor any plateaus. It cannot ever be qualitatively completed. To understand this point is to comprehend the learning role of workers in the process, open to listening and being educated by the oppressed. The vehicle for mutual learning/teaching is dialogue: Dialogue, in turn, is based on trust. According to Freire,

> Trust is contingent on the evidence which one party provides the others of his [sic] true, concrete intentions; it cannot exist if that party's words do not coincide with his [sic] actions. (Freire, 1968, p. 80)

One required component of trust is the ability to communicate one's belief that, despite existing stultified conditions, people have the power to rediscover their capacity to create actively. Dialogue thus implies a relation based on trust, mediated by the concrete, objective world, for the purpose of transforming it: Dialogue is

> The encounter in which the united reflection and action of the dialoguers are addressed to the world which is to be transformed and humanized, [therefore] this dialogue cannot be reduced to the act of one person's 'depositing' ideas in another, nor can it become a simple exchange of ideas to be 'consumed' by the discussants. . . . It is an act of creation; it must not serve as a crafty instrument for the dominantion of one man by another. The domination implicit in dialogue is that of the world by the dialoguers; it is the conquest of the world for the liberation of men [sic]. (Freire, 1968, p. 77)

While dialogue implies an openness to learning and a basic respect for the participants, and trust in them, it also has some preconditions.

In order to respect the oppressed, we must seek to understand the reality they perceive 'so that, knowing it better, [one] can better transform it. [One] is not afraid to confront, to listen, to see the world unveiled' (Freire, 1968, p. 24).

To see the world of the ex-patient as exploitive means to see two dimensions simultaneously: to see profit as extraction from the people with profit-makers as inherently adversaries of the people; and to see how exploited people relate to their conditions. It must be seen critically, in terms of its objective nature, and it must be accepted subjectively as a starting point for action. It also requires seeing domination in two dimensions: objectively, to understand the power relations between landlords or managers, mental health agency staff, etc. and the ex-patient; and to see how the ex-patient expresses him/her self as a reflection of that subjugation. It requires that manipulation be seen in its objective manifestation, in the continuous psychiatric communication of pathology and decompensation; and to see how being coerced into the behavior and ideology of mental illness presents itself as a form of self-expression or as a negotiable identity.

Entering the reality of the ex-patient, a precondition for dialogue, necessitates a dialectical consciousness: a perspective that sees the interpenetration of objective context with subjectivity. It must grasp the contradiction to humanity that the identity of mental patienthood expresses, and accept the given reality as no more than a description of things as they are now, as the beginning of the process of transformation. Freire describes it this way:

> one cannot conceive of objectivity without subjectivity. Neither can exist without the other, nor can they be dichotomized. The separation of objectivity from subjectivity, the denial of the latter when analyzing reality or acting upon it, is objectivism. (Freire, 1968, p. 35)

Objectivism is seen as a world without people; subjectivism, conversely, is people without a world. While these two extremes may seem unreal, our view is that the mental health programs most commonly run are subjectivist in nature, while most of the newer administrative efforts at systematizing mental health planning and management embody objectivist characteristics.

As we have discussed above, the primary theoretical paradigm that has been imposed upon mental patients and ex-patients is medical/ psychopathological in origin. The model is *closed-ended*: the world, the present and the future are circumscribed by a *disease entity* which begins with assumptions about symptoms, extends to remission, and concludes with decompensation. From within the confines of that view, there is simply nowhere to go for the patient or ex-patient, with life posited as an axis having remission and decompensation as its endpoints. This form of thought is called a 'circle of certainty' by Freire who describes such rigid definitions as 'imprisoning reality'. Nothing can enter or leave the closed system, including its purveyors – staff people, as well as patients, being confined in thought and action. It is a static world, having no impetus for change, and no exit. It is exactly this world, supported by the equally closed world of the for-profit, after-care housing facility, that must be seen critically. 'Critical' is used here to connote dialectical consciousness, the totality of relations between objective conditions and subjectivity; between reality as static, 'natural' existence and reality as a historical process requiring intervention. Again, in Freire's words,

> In order for the oppressed to be able to wage the struggle for their liberation, they must perceive the reality of oppression not as a closed world from which there is no exit, but as a limiting situation which they can transform. (Freire, 1968, p. 34)

As discussed above, Dialogue is the vehicle for uncovering the existential reality and opening it to critical reflection. Dialogue cannot be professional interviewing, application of therapeutic technology, instructions for improved functioning or casual conversation. It is purposive in both process and focus. It directs itself to validation of the oppressed as persons, attempting to demonstrate their capacity to inform you, and it struggles to direct the content towards depiction and analysis of the objective situation. This dual purpose initiates the struggle against 'submergence' and lethargy or demoralization, or against objectification. To unveil oppressive reality is to be willing to enter it more fully, to encourage the elaboration of expression, to support the expression of experiences, to initiate the early steps in critical reflection. How and why did/do things happen as they do? How do we know why things unfold as they appear to? Who benefits from current arrangements?

People in oppressed situations, with particularly oppressive histories, often doubt their own validity. This, of course, is rewarding to those benefiting from docility/domination. Both the doubt and self-denial it reproduces are part of the objective context: 'Self-depreciation is another characteristic of the oppressed, which derives from their internalization of the opinion the oppressors hold of them' (Freire, 1968, p. 49). People's self-depreciating subjectivity emerges as part of the objective context to be critically examined, to be construed as a focus for inquiry as to its political content in concealed form.

Professionals in the mental health field, whether from the more traditional disciplines or from the new management programs, almost uniformly are taught to do problem-solving. Most often, the problem-solving process involves gathering information consistent with the professional's or the agency's definition of the problem (see Chapter 1), most often assembling some mechanical procedure and acting on the a priori problem definition, through the agreed upon procedure. This process regulates the world of the professional or agency, forcing the experience of the client/supplicant to 'fit' into a dominated and domesticated reality. Freire suggests another approach: to pose problems to people about their world, 'the organized, systematized and developed "re-presentation" to individuals of the things about which they want to know more' (Freire, 1968, p. 82). Solving a problem, in a conventional sense, ends the discovery of what causes the problem at hand, and others similar to it, to exist. Solving a concrete problem, like getting a Medicaid card, can also be done as a process of posing another one, of looking at the system more broadly than the particular matter at hand. In this latter sense, each issue transcends itself by becoming part of a larger whole: the 'solved problem' of one moment becomes the larger limit-situation to be explored in ongoing dialogue.

Complaining is a commonplace mental patient behavior. In ex-patients confined to facilities of one type or another, whining about food, money, toilet paper, unheated rooms, etc. is a way of life. What they say is rarely listened to, because they are the ones saying it – their comments about their environment and their way of presenting themselves are seen as part of their pathology. Complaining presents itself as entirely subjective, and most often is dismissed or used by service workers or management as the substance for ridicule. Where the resident persists or changes the form of expression, the behavior is often seen as 'acting out.'

Seeing a complaint as a disguised or concealed critical comment, however, allows the possibility of taking both the disguise and the issue differently. Taken seriously, the whining must give way to the person taking responsibility for further elaboration, discussion about why the situation is as it is, etc. What exactly is the complaint about? How can the two or more of you explore it in greater detail? Why is the situation as it is? Who benefits? A complaint is transformed into a research process of mutual investigation. Questions can often initiate dialogue far better than answers – the ex-patient is legitimated as a critical commentator about his/her situation at the same time as the passivity of the complaint is elevated to an issue on which some type of action can be taken. This, in turn, poses the form of expression as a problem. As the complaint becomes objectively received, the object/ex-patient is encouraged to elaborate and to share what she/he knows with peers and is supported to extend questioning and assessing. To the extent that the limits of the situation can be explored and mutually documented (an objective base), the action stance of the ex-patient can move from inevitable passive adaptation to one of strategic contemplation. In most instances, over time, complaints about the home become criticisms of owners or managers, and strategies for acting on the issue present the profit-makers as objectively existing adversaries of the residents, a major shift in perception which withdraws or denies vital legitimation from oppressors.

When Freire says that oppressed people are aware that they are downtrodden, but their perception of themselves is impaired by the objective reality that submerges them, he means that people's feelings about their situation have no basis in conventional conceptual validation, and thus their perceptions are experienced as both subjective and distorted. People's feelings about the owners of the places where they have been deposited, for example, are clouded, mystified or devalued because owners or managers are frequently included as part of aftercare treatment teams by mental health and social services workers. Power and legitimation are fused in this odd marriage: the owners of mental health and the owners of the facility join together, leaving ex-patients no power base or viability structure to provide conceptual legitimacy to their experience. The conceptual machinery that is both observable and operative is as out of control of the ex-patients as is their objective condition. Self-denigration, in the form of whining behavior and taken for granted complaints, reproduces the situation entirely.

Dialogue, which takes both the person and the content of his/her self-expression seriously, introduces problems into the context for both the ex-patient and for the mental health or social services worker and the owners. Problems break the omnipresent static atmosphere of management and conventional treatment by holding both up to critical reflection and responsive action. Quite obviously, just, fair, objectively legitimate providers need have no fear since their participation would emerge with a more authentic validation.

Part of recognizing the experiential dimension of submergence requires comprehending its omnipotence. Whether enmeshed in the medical or psycho-social rehabilitation approaches, clear-cut contours exist as boundaries to former patients' behaviors and consciousness. Permissible behaviors or consciousness are shaped by mental patient social role structures and reproduce mental patient identity (and, therefore, reproduce staff identity). Whether the desired outcome is docile maintenance or quantitatively improved functioning, or both, the circle of behavior-consciousness-behavior is closed: it can go nowhere except back to reinforcing itself and the social context which created it. It is a fixed world which parallels the circle of certainty governing the thought structure of the models it represents. Confined to static existence, relegated to consume coercively services designed to obstruct human development through improving mental patient functioning, former patients are locked in very much as they were while living on closed wards. Having learned the psychiatric world view, any negative feelings experienced as a reflection of the objective context are joined immediately by contradicting feelings of fear of decompensation and of being rehospitalized.

Transformation requires reconnection to the objective world of daily oppression. Subjective validation occurs only through this process of rehumanization, of becoming a participant in producing the social world. But this process must be initiated by those not so fully submerged, by those capable of critical reflection about exploitation, domination and manipulation. This act of leadership, of teaching, begins with the effort to identify aspects of the 'no exit' reality which can be contemplated. Freire refers to this engagement activity as limit-setting or problem-posing: the task is to identify some area of daily life about which former patients have a concern, usually voiced as a complaint. The purpose is to reflect on whatever topic is presented in order to show its base in social reality: to reduce it from the inevitable to social historical fact.

Identification of topics for opening dialogue requires that workers know the entire array of legal rights, entitlements and benefits available to former patients (see Chapter 6) because these factors often form baselines for reference as responses to complaints. They also can form the basis for an 'intake' interview and/or 'assessment' procedure in which the message is that the concrete conditions of daily life are central to well-being. In any event, the purpose is to stimulate discourse concerning some aspect of everyday life perceived by the former patient as simultaneously omnipresent, inevitable, beyond change. Its subject-specific content can either be the former patient him/herself in relation to his/her concept of his/her own identity or some facet of the context which reproduces that identity. The focus of the exchange is to develop a process of *elaboration* of the perception of the ex-patient, of what she/he perceives, of how she/he came to see it that way, of how she or he see themselves, and of why they see things as they do. According to Freire, discussion of whatever the topic may be is purposive:

> that which had existed objectively but had not been perceived in its deeper implication (if indeed it was perceived at all) begins to 'stand out', assuming the character of a problem and therefore of challenge. Thus, men [sic] begin to single out elements from their 'background awarenesses' and to reflect upon them. (Freire, 1968, p. 70)

As this process begins, people may learn to see their reality as somewhat permeable through their own reflection and action.

Background awareness, as Freire calls it, refers to what people know about their situations, but have no reason to validate or believe to be true. People's views of their own perception generally correspond to their own sense of their validity as observers. The process of becoming a mental patient and remaining a former patient has stripped most people of their sense of validity. The objective context, coupled with medical language and thought structures, has reduced and distorted people's validity and legitimacy as participants in perceiving and acting in their own behalf. They are coerced into consuming the social reality of domination in much the same way they consume medication – as passive receptacles, relatively powerless to resist in a confrontation with their situation.

Ironically, the only time they are seen as capable of making decisions is when they resist by refusing to continue taking medication, an acting out, a 'symptom' of decompensation. Consuming reality, and therefore reproducing it, consists of accepting the situation as it is – without the 'deeper implications' or causes of that reality, in Freire's terms. Reflection on reality, and one's experience in it, can be initiated through dialogue, through reflection based on identification of generative themes and limit-setting or problem-posing communication designed to transform 'background awarenesses' to their deeper implications, the preconditions for action. Through this process, which we discuss below, people reflecting on their social world also reflect on themselves in that world, as part of that world. This, in turn, will alter the parameters for action since the form or type of action people are willing to take 'is to a large extent a function of how they perceive themselves in the world' (Freire, 1968, p. 71).

The point of intervention must be the interface between the situation that people find themselves in and their perception of themselves in that situation. According to Freire, 'Only by starting from this situation – which determines their perception of it – can they begin to move' (1968, p. 73). Since the situation constitutes the living arrangements and service consuming activities of the ex-patient, a dramatic irony presents itself: the very reality which the homeowners and service providers want to be taken for granted (if not adored) becomes the focus of inquiry. That which the 'stabilizers' or purveyors of maintenance therapy want obscured becomes the focal point for observation and the starting point for critical reflection. The purpose is to transform that which is perceived as both omnipotent and inevitable into that which is social, historical and alterable.

The possibilities for initiating dialogue in the world of the ex-patient are infinite: anything dealing with money can lead to discussions of where cheques come from or how mail is handled, what the law and regulations say about benefits, about the contractual (as opposed to 'therapeutic') relation to landlords, etc. Similarly, simple inquiry into typical mental health and/or health care can introduce reflection about how the ex-patient is perceived: what do they know about their own care, about the medication(s) prescribed, about side effects, about their rights to know what is happening to them? In each case, whatever the focus of discussion, the purpose is to have the person elaborate on the social reality that they perceive and to introduce into the discourse the validity of people's feelings about what they have described as well as to elicit their observations about why things exist as they do.

The process of dialogue, described in part here, therefore contributes to several dimensions simultaneously. It develops the action of dialectical social reality – what exists objectively relates directly to what is experienced subjectively, either in a logically consistent form or a contradictory one. Where contradictions exist between the 'supposed to' version of reality and the experienced account, the issue of whose interests are served or who benefits and in what way becomes a focus of inquiry. Dialogue also develops validation: the former patient is central to the discourse as a person (versus mental patient) whose observations make sense, even though they may be objectively incorrect. Where the sense is submerged in the reality of oppression, the dialogue seeks to investigate the causes of oppression, again using the theme of interests served by existing conditions. Action possibilities, involving people in making strategic choices about their lives, or aspects of their lives, represent the beginning of transformation from consumer/reproducer to participant/producer of the process of living.

In order to participate in the type of dialogue we have been discussing, workers must assume responsibility for actively knowing what ex-patients' lives involve – to see where they live and learn how they see it; to visit the day program or vocational rehabilitation center and learn what they think about it and how it feels to be there; to visit the hospitals and clinics to learn their meanings. Through inviting discussion about these broad areas of life, dialogue can be initiated as an open-ended process based on persons communicating – rather than on patients consuming therapy.

In the struggle to initiate dialogue, we must remember what the people have been through in their life histories – periods of total institutionalization and dehumanization. The social identity of the mental patient, supported as it is by landlords and mental health programs, will most often produce a scepticism about other workers who profess a different orientation. Breaking through the barriers of coercive history is a long, arduous task. It requires building trust based on activity or actual differences in the content and process of dialogue. Since so much of the people's daily life bears more resemblance to daily life in the hospital than to a more liberating social existence, we must remember the obstacles and potential threats that are posed by interaction with others (like us) who present a critical consciousness, no matter how benignly we may appear. To see and accept the people as they are is a beginning point, not a permanent determination. Freire expresses it this way:

> The starting point for organizing the program content of [intervention] must be the present, existential, concrete situation, reflecting the aspirations of the people. Utilizing certain basic contradictions, we must pose this existential, concrete, present situation to the people as a problem which challenges them and requires a response – not just at the intellectual level, but at the level of action. (Freire, 1968, p. 85)

Hopefully, we understand that reaching the decision to act is a momentous one, not to be confused with verbiage that connotes tacit acquiescence to what we communicate as our expectations. This would be yet another accommodating adaptation to power.

Freire is well aware of potential tendencies of workers towards imposing their views on the oppressed, and seeing in acquiescence a more genuine response. We are warned about the negation of our beliefs that such action would precipitate:

> It is not our role to speak to the people about our own view of the world, nor to attempt to impose that view on them, but rather to dialogue with the people about their view and ours. We must realize that their view of the world, manifested variously in their action, reflects their situation in the world. (Freire, 1968, p. 85)

We express our view through our actions as well, not in lectures or presentations of sophisticated analyses, but in questions and solicitations about their world and their view of it that allow them to elaborate – as persons – on their perceptions. And it is our responsibility to pose problems about aspects of concrete daily life that are presently accepted by ex-patients as a reflection of their situation (as permanent conditions). It is not our task to win people over, to have them accept our view: 'After all,' Freire says, 'the task of humanists is surely not that of pitting their slogans against the slogans of the oppressors, with the oppressed as the testing ground. . . .' (1968, p. 84).

Accepting these premises suggests a major change for many mental health workers. In the past, the nature of questions raised has focused on a linear concept of subjectivity – inquiring about how people (really, about patients) feel, and presuming that feelings registered symptom states rather than reflecting objective conditions. Mental health workers have also had great difficulty seeing present, existential status as permeable or capable of transformation since medical diagnoses of mental illness tend to presuppose a permanent condition which may fluctuate somewhat, but never be transformed. In this regard, training of these workers must itself change dramatically, and in accordance with the same principles they will be asked to utilize in their work with ex-patients. This suggests that simple transfer of new information, or mandated new language, without sufficient exploration of the workers' view of the world will be self-defeating.* It is

---

* See 'You Catch More Flies With Honey Than With Vinegar. . . .', a critical study of mental health workers' responses to legal advocacy training, by Diane Johnson *et al.* (1982).

exactly in the exploration of the workers' social world and their perception of it that some identification with their ex-patient clients can be built. This occurs because the workers, too, contend with fiscal crisis, the stressful relations between people that arise from it, and from their prior work experience, all of which must be analyzed critically.

We emphasize this point because we have experienced frequent frustration from seeing transparent domination and exploitation of ex-patients, particularly by landlords, responded to 'passively.' We put quotation marks around this last word to indicate that its usage is condemning, a failure to enter the reality of long term coercion and adaptive response. Our survival and/or development strategy usually has some type of 'progress' built into it rather than acquiescence, but that reflects our social historical situation, just as the response of ex-patients reflects their dialectical connection to the reality they have endured. The challenge to workers is not to solve the problems posed by this situation alone – or even to try, unless the situation were life threatening. Rather, the task is to recognize the apparent contradiction and to take responsibility for creating a way to make the obvious turn into a problematic situation for the ex-patient. This requires knowing more about how the person thinks and speaks than is ever required in conventional practice because our task is not to become the problem to the person, but rather to have some aspect of their reality become conscious as an area of potential activity directed toward change. This requires that the ex-patient(s) see a major change – that what they have perceived as impermeable becomes comprehensible as capable of being changed.

Identifying proper issues is a difficult task, one that does not lend itself to liberal outrage. We have found that the best method for locating issues is to be fully aware of the entire array of legal rights and entitlements that pertain to former patients' lives. Legislation, policy decisions, regulations, guidelines and court decisions all exist in such daily life matters as landlord-tenant relations, licensing and regulating agencies for facilities of one kind or another, Medicaid, SSI, etc. Thorough familiarity with this material can allow workers to see transgressions by homeowners or agencies and to introduce the disparity into the ongoing dialogue. It helps to have the material at hand, and to have it in some simplified language, perhaps in the form of a booklet to share with clients (see Taichman *et al.*, 1980a and 1980b). Once people know that their entitlements have been violated, and that there is some body of law and advocacy behind them, their readiness to contemplate action can change. We do want to stress, however, that the decision to act must always rest with the client. Simply putting law or policy before them, apart from the ongoing relationship and struggle towards dialogue, will either terminate contact or produce a double bind which the worker imposes. Trying to find the balance between our own desire and need to produce change, and the support needed by clients to move in a similar direction is a delicate matter. For it to become part of an ongoing process, and not a situation of our 'winning' compliance from them, we can constantly remember that the decision must be theirs, that we can pose the issue of probable implications for them for each potential action, and we can be clear about where and when they can count on us for support, and in what ways. Whatever the decision,the aftermath will affect the ex-patient in a different way than it will affect the worker, and it is the worker who must keep this fact in mind.

Summary

In this chapter we have tried to articulate a set of practice principles which move from the overriding theoretical perspective of the Introduction through the intermediate theory level (problem definition) to practice. As we move on, our task will be to discuss the application of these principles in both direct practice settings and in 'indirect' practice. Because we see intervention strategies deriving from an analysis of the context in relation to problem definition, and therefore dynamic (or alive to change, open to information and experience, not capable of complete anticipation), we have been careful not to call our approach a model. We do this purposefully to suggest to the readers their own creative responsibility for design and application of the principles discussed above. Quite obviously, a 'model' for practice places primary focus on a pre-existing external mechanical procedure(s), with the person involved as secondary, and the target population as tertiary. Our approach or design cannot make this bureaucratically convenient and comfortable somersault for it would stand reality on its head. Our beginning point must be the context – historical and social – which forms the contours for people's lives.

Taking this position involves a different set of expectations for workers – rather than being able to rely on professional training and socialization into structured roles, workers must be able to resist the parameters of expression that such roles impose, and risk opening themselves to the situations they encounter as people who have taken particular jobs to survive. We emphasize this point because the structured roles of the vast majority of agencies do not have the open-ended potential for learning from client groups. More typically, they confine both workers and target populations to predetermined understandings (perhaps labels) which serve to justify intervention models and agency procedures at the expense of the people served, and the workers.

Allowing ourselves to enter the reality of the people with whom we work, and to do so critically, requires that we comprehend the objective historical circumstances people confront. Often such knowledge is bypassed in professional education where theories and analytical methods usually rationalize the institutions and professions as part of the process of socializing neophytes into a tradition. Since, most often, these very institutions and professions are not seen as positive influences in people's lives, workers struggling to create an advocacy/empowerment design will have to experience some distance from their training and often from their employers. This is no mean chore, but must be contemplated and critically reflected upon in ongoing work, using much the same approach taken with client groups – a critical reflection of the objective circumstances and their influence on subjective experience.

Being open to learning from clients is unfamiliar. Often, being open to hearing information outside the boundaries of one's training is unknown, since a major aspect of professional indoctrination involves categorizing what one hears, especially if one hears it from those identified as clients. For those clients having had extensive experience with workers, a similar situation may pertain. The challenge to us, as workers, is a difficult one – to continue to encourage people to elaborate on their perceptions and the causes for their perceptions, without making clinical judgments and without reacting defensively. It may even require accepting one's own lack of validity and searching for its objective historical basis.

And, finally, one has to confront a most difficult perception: the social world of the people we work with is indeed objectively characterized by oppression, domination and manipulation. In our experience, workers may seem to understand these terms rhetorically, but deny their concrete existence. To do this turns objective historical conditions into subjectivity, a demeaning practice for both clients and workers. It serves only the class privilege of the workers, the only ones free to leave the conditions behind at the end of each working day. It also allows workers to believe that conflicts such as must arise in the struggle for freedom can be resolved through some process of rational agreement.

We turn now to an elaboration of advocacy/empowerment practice expressed as a social action strategy. In the next chapter we attempt to integrate problem definition theory with advocacy/empowerment practice principles.

The chapters which comprise Section II attempt to demonstrate the viability of the advocacy/empowerment design in several different types of setting and forms of practice. These descriptions are not meant to be blueprints for others to follow, but serve instead to exemplify the practice principles drawn from Freire. They are an attempt to initiate a dialogue, rather than conclude one, to stimulate creativity rather than curtail it. We hope to demonstrate that the principles applied to the target population, in the specific circumstances where we work, have positive impact on both clients and workers. Since elements of the situation are common in many areas, aspects of how we have chosen to function may apply to other situations as well. In any case, we present them as an invitation to readers to critically reflect on their own practice and to join the creative enterprise of designing their own tasks, hoping that the theoretical framework presented above provides a valid conceptual orientation to organizing intervention strategies.

CHAPTER 3

Towards an Advocacy/Empowerment Action Orientation

Converting practice principles into action is clearly not a random activity. As we demonstrate in the practice chapters which follow this section of the book, our concept of practice contains a theory of social action. It is the task of this chapter to describe the advocacy/ empowerment action orientation which guides our work. As a preamble to this discussion, however, we want to make two transcending assumptions: that a guide for action is not a map, a set of concretized standards, or a maze through which one must travel according to a set prescription; and that the course of action will be as necessarily determined by the actors involved as is its overriding purposes, that the people always transcend the means they choose to express their interests.

Any program or agency committed to an advocacy/empowerment action orientation asserts that one of the most critical needs of human beings is the need to be a creative and effective participant in one's environment. We made this point earlier when we distinguished between being a participating creator in one's daily life rather than functioning only as a consumer of it (see Navarro, 1983, on the fallacy of consumption as a viable basis of power and legitimation). To act in and upon the social world and to struggle to transform it, thus creating ever new possibilities for expressing one's individual and collective interests, is what Freire refers to as our species-specific 'ontological vocation' (Freire, 1968). This belief implies that an advocacy/ empowerment action orientation also sees the human being, regardless of previous dehumanization, exploitation, domination, or mystification (i.e., deinstitutionalized former psychiatric patients), potentially capable of critical intervention into his or her reality.

Seeing the person as a potentially active agent in the process of creating the social world suggests that the experience of expressing one's human interests occurs not only in reacting to existing objective conditions, but in acting as a subject on those conditions and consciously struggling to transform them. Since the social world is created out of the interaction of human subjectivity and objective historical conditions, people acting to transform oppressive conditions which only reproduce their situation are simultaneously acting to transform themselves. The social world, in the process of its development, consists of the interacting 'known' circumstances and persons 'known' as allocated social roles, and 'knowing' subjects acting to create a more liberated possibility for human experience and expression. The particular expression of this objective-subjective interaction, at a microsocial level, is mediated by the way in which the people participating in the struggle see themselves in their world. Put another way, the self-concept of the persons involved in the exigencies of daily life contours the way people participate in it. When one's self-concept is ridden with externally imposed contempt, when a person incorporates the devalued perception of his or her oppressors, and acts through that self-concept in the social world, the result will inevitably be the reproduction of the objective conditions dominated by oppressive interests. We believe this to be the common, shared experience of daily life for most former psychiatric patients.

An advocacy/empowerment action orientation rejects medicalized models of treatment because they sever the interactional relation between objective reality (economic, social, political, legal and ideological structures) and subjective reality (self-concept, perception, emotional life). Medicalized practice and implied action schemes overemphasize either the objective side (the pure medical model which sees the person as a medical entity or object) *or* the subjective (emotional) dimension of the relationship and ignore the objective side, thus distorting the dialectical, interpenetrating, emergent character of social reality or human action. The subjectivist distortion reflects a skewed understanding of the problems of ex-patients, and in the formulations of solutions to those false problems which exclude ex-patients from meaningful participation in daily life by robbing them of their legitimation as potentially active agents in their own behalf. Operating within the medicalized paradigm of practice reduces human potential to the confines of drugs and mental patient role reproducing programs, thus short-circuiting social development and reproducing the conditions of oppression. This type of treatment thus constitutes a downward spiral wherein objective conditions reinforce dehumanized subjective expression (mental patient roles) which, in turn, reproduce the circumstances of domination. Medicalized forms of practice thus effectively bar or deny former patients participation in the construction of their own lives and reduce them to consumers of the lives determined for them by others.

In contrast to the unidirectional practices criticized here, an advocacy/empowerment action orientation emphasizes a dialectical interactionist perspective which better captures the complexity of the social world of deinstitutionalized former psychiatric patients. This view enables us to formulate strategies which respond to both the objective-social and subjective-psychological dimensions of need expressed in this population. A strategy with dual focus is required to confront the vicious cycle of oppressive conditions reproducing alienated subjective conditions (the downward spiral). One focus of the advocacy/empowerment strategy is to develop direct service program relationships with ex-patients. It is to promote individual and collective struggle to understand and transform concrete problems in daily life through a process of trust, validation, support, legitimation and action designed to produce alteration in self-concept concomitant with changing degrees of autonomy and control. (These matters are developed in discussions of two common areas of practice in Chapters 4 and 5.) The other focus involves advocacy activities designed to change objective conditions beyond the immediate situations endured by most ex-patients (these activities are presented in Chapters 6, 7 and 8).

As we move toward development of an action orientation in the realm of direct practice, to restore the objective-subjective dialectic to former patients, we must recall the necessity of avoiding two pitfalls in daily practice. These include the abandonment of leadership responsibility and the contrasting tendency towards over-direction or domination. Either of these two tendencies can arise as easily understandable reactions to either the objective conditions of daily life thrust upon most ex-patients (more likely to produce over-direction toward some action against landlords, for example), and/or reaction to mental patient identity, the form of social existence thrust upon ex-patients by mental health treatment (more likely to produce denial of leadership and pseudo-therapeutic passivity). Where the more activist pitfall threatens to place ex-patients in jeopardy as well as to continue their

domination (albeit by other, more 'pure' hands), the abandonment
pitfall reproduces the domination and oppression of ex-patients by
presuming their difficulties to be subjective and responsive to therapeutic encounters. This latter and more common error (another
instance of Freire's concept of 'false charity') derives from the failure
to understand the totality of domination contained in the mental
patient identity. In failing to recognize the self-contempt required by
socialization into mental patient roles and identity, the therapeutic
mental health perspective functions to reproduce the conditions of
domination in a 'charitable' way. Naive subjectivism recreates the
same problems as naive activism; the ex-patients remain dominated
and submerged in a reality controlled by others.

The central problem to be addressed by an advocacy/empowerment
action scheme is to identify ways in which an oppressed, alienated and
mystified population can participate in a struggle directed toward
increased conscious autonomy and dignity. How can workers engaging
in an advocacy/empowerment practice avoid validating mental
patient-like behavior, while at the same time avoid manipulating the
people toward the workers' own objectives? More concretely, how can
workers in direct practice settings encourage ex-patients not to choose
the activities and areas of engagement reflective of their socialization
into mental patient roles and identities (a false choice created by
refusal to acknowledge ex-patients' prior exploitation and mode of
adaptation to it)? Or avoid a situation where 'doing anything else
meant continuing the manipulation and domination by obscuring it'
(Rose and Chaglasian, 1978, p. 56).

The advocacy/empowerment action scheme

What is the process by which one enters into the reality of the
ex-patient, understands and learns from that reality, and validates the
person communicating his or her experience, yet simultaneously
provides leadership directed toward critical appraisal of what one has
heard? The purpose of the advocacy/empowerment action orientation
is to produce change or movement of the deinstitutionalized former
patient from a position of passive powerlessness and self-destructive
alienation to one of increased self-conscious autonomy through implementation of a series of action phrases. While these phases are
delineated as distinct entities in Figure 3.1 – the Advocacy/

1 *Verstehen*
   a learning from ex-patients
   b grasping the essance of the subjective meanings of ex-patients
   c preliminary presentation of alternative construction of social reality via legal rights and entitlements

2 *Thematization*
   a alienation
      – exploitation
      – powerlessness
      – isolation
      – dependence
   b submergence
      – world as natural fact
      – mystified about oppression
      – fatalism
      – self-contempt

3 *Problematization*
   a legal rights and entitlements
   b validation of *person* vs. mental patient
   c validation/leadership
   d world as problem to be solved

4 *Anomie*
   normlessness
   confusion
   anxiety
   anger
   fear

5 *Analysis of the consequences of action*
   a Objective meaning
      – possible retaliation
      – possible success/failure
      – individual vs. collective action
   b patient role to personal appearance

6 *Choice*
   a decisions made by ex-patient
   b 'never sacrifice a person for an issue'

7 *Action*
   a informed participation
   b collective struggle
   c inter-organization advocacy

8 *Evaluation*
   a observe consequences of action
      – plan for next action
   b Subjective meaning
      – self-concept as participant vs. adaptor
      – self-concept as strategist vs. consumer

Verstehen
   a learning from each other
   b learning qua social being
   c grasping the essence of objective oppression
   d grasping the meaning of conflict and the need for strategic engagment

Figure 3.1

Empowerment Action Scheme – the entire action orientation is perceived to be a process of mutual interaction between ex-patients and workers, provoked by the objective conditions of domination in daily life and their subjective counterparts in the experience and self-concept of the ex-patient population *and* by the leadership activities of the advocacy/empowerment oriented workers who are guided by the problem definition (discussed above in Chapter 1) and the practice principles discussed in Chapter 2. The transcending commitment to this *interactive process* requires that the phases outlined below be understood primarily as heuristic devices rather than as mechanical, empirically related entities which supersede the interactions of the involved participants.

As the Action Scheme is examined, we ask that the reader attempt to picture it as circular, with each set of arrows pointing in multiple directions to indicate that the dimensions of action interact with one another in various ways, many of which are not predictable, and none of which are fixed or predetermined as 'the proper way' to engage in an advocacy/empowerment practice. We hope that this visual presentation of the elements of action will clarify our advocacy/empowerment action scheme and provide a useful perspective on the implementation of the practice principles discussed above.

Verstehen, the first phase, is a process of developing a 'sympathetic understanding' of the subjective meanings former patients have of themselves and their situations. It includes coming to understand the ex-patient's self-concept as the center of his or her perception of the universe of daily experience, of his or her view of his or her own needs, goals or aspirations as well as of frustrations and pain. As part of the process of *Verstehen*, the worker pieces together the ex-patient's use of language, the connection between language and its reference points (perceived by going with the client to the various places that the client uses to locate daily life experience, for example, the adult home or SRO where the client lives, the rehabilitation program where the client spends weekdays or the continuing treatment program or mental health clinic, etc.), and the meanings of these objective circumstances and conditions in the ex-patient's life. Dialogue, as discussed in Chapter 2, is the medium of exchange for this learning process. It is a vehicle for mutual communication, for as the worker learns from the client what he or she needs to know about the client, and the world of client-centered perception and experience, the client is simultaneously learning about a different type of mental health worker, about a person who wants to know rather than about a person who wants to instruct, or coerce or neglect. The combination of continuous efforts at eliciting elaboration from the client about his or her perception and experience, together with the initial introduction of relevant rights and entitlements data to the client, is the building block for plausibility – for combining new words and ideas with new experiences to allow for critical examination of the reality of daily life, with a view towards changing it.

Thematization, the second phase of our action scheme, is dependent upon the worker's success at elaboration with clients. From clients' extended descriptive accounts of their world of experience and self-concepts, we identify the lived existence of 'generative themes.' These themes are the more broad-based objective conditions and subjective reflections of those conditions expressed through the lives of the former patients, but hidden from their conscious awareness by the prevailing oppression and its mystification (e.g., landlords as members of treatment teams, mental health workers not cognizant or even interested in transparently oppressive living conditions, etc.). It is through *Verstehen* and its commitment to elaboration that the prevailing themes in their distorted understanding are made known and later used to redefine problems of a more particular scope (whining or complaining about food or living conditions is transformed into serious criticisms of housing, which in turn is reflexively seen as exploitation via extended discussion of the owner as landlord and the 'bond' between ex-patient and owner as a lease rather than a treatment plan).

Two of the salient 'generative themes' for an advocacy/empowerment action orientation are alienation and submergence. These two themes reflect the two related realms within the totality of oppressive existence for most ex-patients. Alienation reflects the poverty, exploitation, domination and powerless isolation imposed upon ex-patients through both the objective conditions of everyday life and by the coercively dependent behaviors imprinted upon mental patient identity. Submergence, as the dialectically related dimension, reflects the legitimation given to the oppression and its concomitant mystification of reality. Included in the concept of submergence is a perception of the world as permanent and closed, as a 'natural fact' that cannot be changed. Submergence also connotes a mystification about the sources of the problems confronted and their legitimation; as such, it is characterized by adaptivity or conformity, fatalism and self-contempt.

Problematization, or the third phase in the advocacy/empowerment action scheme, comes about as a result of the leadership of the workers. It reflects the abilities of the workers to thematize the elaborated descriptive material presented to them by their ex-patient clients, to represent to the former patients in a critical fashion the material given to the workers in a non-critical descriptive form, and the capacity of the workers to partialize or to frame thematically defined problems in interim level or actionable level terms. Using the larger themes that reflect the daily life situations of ex-patients critically, problems are formulated out of what was previously accepted as given and natural (fixed and unchangeable). Problematization presents an irreconcilable conflict to the closed, 'given' world expressed through and by mental patient identity and through the 'normal' relationships of former patients and their 'caretakers'. It presents problems to be solved where previously there were none; it presents the world as contingent upon human action rather than as static and independent of social existence; and it transforms the fatalism felt in everyday life into a restored capacity to act. As these openings began to appear in ex-patients' perceptions of the objective world, so too will there appear openings in the subjective realm of self-concept and experienced feelings about oneself in the world.

The provision of information about legal rights and entitlements, on a regular basis, and directly in response to complaints about objective conditions, is a recurring way to problematize ex-patients' objective reality. At a descriptive level of everyday language, it may involve constant reference to the homeowner as landlord, thus suggesting an altered relationship from the treatment team mentality of the other service providers. Another example might include referring to ex-patients' legal right to hold their own Medicaid card or choose their own physician. At the same time, relating to ex-patients as human beings with legitimate concerns, and thus with the dignity that status deserves, problematizes the ex-patients' subjective reality. The experiencing of oneself as a passive mental patient is made more difficult when others relate to a person as an active human being. Over a period of time, when either the objective or subjective dimensions of reality are problematized, what previously has been experienced as 'natural', and requiring no choice, can emerge as requiring participation and action of some type. It becomes increasingly problematic for former patients to view the existing situation as unchanging 'natural fact.' The discovery by ex-patients that reality has a dimension of choice and participation opens up previously held and felt perceptions about both the reality of everyday life and one's place within it. It makes available to consciousness the possibility for intervention into reality.

Anomie, the fourth phase of the advocacy/empowerment action scheme, depicts a period in which the ex-patient, who has been able to engage in dialogue, to elaborate his or her thoughts and feelings about the experience of everyday life, responds to the thematization provided by workers in order to problematize reality, and endures a situation in which he or she does not constantly relate to any fixed set of norms or guideposts for comprehending everyday life. This situation arises as one comes to see and believe that one's life situation is different from what one had previously been coerced into believing it was, and that things do not have to be the way they have been. Experientially, we have seen this phase expressed in clients as confusion, fear, anxiety or anger, feelings previously buried in the interpenetration of mental patient identity and intensity-deadening medications. The upsurge of any of these feelings, when coupled with the ambiguity in conceptual frameworks provoked by being taken seriously as a human being, often produces intense fear of recurring 'symptoms' and of 'decompensation.' The strong remnants of the mental patient identity, accumulated over years of 'treatment,' lead to the fear that the person is becoming mentally ill again, that the valid subjective reflection of the ex-patients' true situation is really the re-emergence of their sickness. This period thus requires continuous contact and rapid follow-up should appointments be missed or attendance at day programs slack off, and anticipation of needed validation and support. The ex-patients must have readily available some honest, critical source of support for the fact that their experience is valid, understandable, and readily identifiable as deriving from their objective circumstances. Ex-patients are urged not to determine present actions based on the immediacy of intense feelings of anger or rage, nor on the automatic suspension of action that such feelings have produced in prior years. As an alternative, and further incentive to their own development, the people are encouraged to share their situation and feelings with workers and peers, to think through what problem situations specifically require their most immediate attention, and what potential consequences of action possibilities or tactics exist for each targeted area of concern.

Analysis of the consequences of action, the fifth phase of the advocacy/empowerment action scheme, is required as part of the process of strategic contemplation of action. This phase implies that the ex-patient has learned something starkly divergent from his or her previously perceived reality; that a conflict of interest exists between him or her and several important people, including homeowners and management, physician or perhaps psychiatrists or other mental health personnel – the 'gatekeepers' who have created or reinforced mental patient identity and personal submergence. The immediate, non-strategic expression of rage or frustration toward a landlord is a sure predictor of rehospitalization and continued invalidation. What recent experience does the ex-patient have in thinking strategically, or in thinking of him or herself as a strategist? Lengthy deliberation is required to figure out which actions to take on objective conditions, if any, as well as to reflect on oneself as a strategic thinking and planning person. The more subjective aspect of this phase functions as a support for the person familiarizing him or herself anew with the basic dignity inherent in being a socially human being rather than an asocial mental patient-object. Central to the analytic process described here is an acknowledgment of power and interest differentials existent in the situation. With this recognition comes the beginning of the transformation from adaptive, objectified consumer of others' reality to the position of active participant, chooser of one's own preferred way of being in the world.

Choice, the sixth phase of the advocacy/empowerment action scheme, like the others, contains both an objective and subjective dimension. The objective aspect is found in the selection of an action stance vis-à-vis whatever target has been determined as the focus for intervention (including the choice not to act in the present, but to sustain the process of analysis of a situation for the time being). The subjective aspects involves the person reflecting on him or herself as a choice-maker, as an active, creative participant. Essential to this phase is a principle of advocacy/empowerment practice – never is a person to be sacrificed for an issue. Concretely, workers must struggle to ensure that ex-patients are not coerced or made to feel compelled into acting on an issue to satisfy the needs or feelings of workers. The vulnerable position of the ex-patient, the jeopardy involved (to them) from acting on an issue is the focus of the matter, not the subjective needs of the worker. This requires that a decision not to take action in any given situation be respected as a strategic choice, rather than denigrated as cowardly or unwise. When the focus of objective action is defined as a choice for non-action, the decision must be validated and supported. This can more easily be understood by workers when the issue of the subjective development of the person is again put forward as equally vital activity to more readily observable changes in the objective sector. In the situation where the choice has been made to refrain from action in the present situation, the advocacy/empowerment activities required stress the process of the person-as-participant, of the immense growth that is represented in the person-as-strategist when compared to the person previously seen as mental patient. The issue is slightly altered to focus on the submergence-consciousness dimension and the tremendous courage displayed by the ex-patient engaging in a dialogue with potentially threatening outcomes. This throws the focus back onto conditions in the objective world and allows the person to continue to be validated for the process of struggle rather than simply to be praised for measurable outcomes.

Action, the seventh phase of the advocacy/empowerment action scheme, is already underway in the analysis of the consequences phase. Its focus is on the informed, conscious participation on the part of ex-patients throughout the planning and carrying out of any action. The advocacy/empowerment action orientation will not 'do for' the ex-patients, nor does it call for abandoning them to fend for themselves. It provides information and support for self-conscious, informed participation, critical reflection on the potential ramifications of various choices, and validation for the people engaged in the situation. It may also require critical refusal, in those instances where the action strategy being enacted suggests that potential danger or harm that is not understood will be the prevailing by-product of the action (for example, when a person's rage at the circumstances imposed upon him or her by a landlord overwhelms the capacity to think strategically and the person strikes out against other ex-patients sharing the same housing).

Evaluation, the eighth phase of the action scheme, is necessary in order to continue the process of personal development and intervention into objective circumstances. To observe what has been accomplished, and to reflect on the experience of taking collective action or individual initiative, and to base further action upon critical reflection and shared experience is the brick and mortar of continued social development, of developing increased autonomy, dignity and community. In any evaluative process, both objective and subjective dimensions of the activity must be reviewed. This allows for critical discussion of the value of any given tactic or action choice, while concomitantly promoting the validation of the participants. Advocacy/empowerment-oriented workers must pay special attention to this subjective aspect of practice since ex-patients, individually and collectively, have so little experience perceiving themselves to be legitimate, active, producers of at least some part of their everyday reality. Support for the continuous shift from consumer of conventional mental health services and consumer of the service providers' reality to sharing in the production of their own version of objective reality (rather than subjective reality, the reduced realm of submerged being for all mental patients) thus emerges as a major practice component of the evaluative phase.

With the completion of the advocacy/empowerment action scheme, both the workers and the clients find themselves at another beginning. *Verstehen*, however, takes on a somewhat different meaning: as the client-participants engage in the process of dialogue directed toward action to change oppressive reality, they become changed themselves in the process of the struggle. They experience themselves with decreasing self-contempt, and with less contempt for others who have shared their experience and their demeaned social status; they feel more dignity subjectively; they more readily contemplate legal rights and entitlements and more readily initiate problematized perspectives on problems confronting them. These expressions of development, however minute they may appear, must be supported. As the participants experience themselves more legitimately, as their role in dialogue changes, the circle of participants in it grows, and the possibilities for expanded collective action change to reflect the other realms of growth.

Conclusion

The advocacy/empowerment action orientation contends that a dialectical interactionist view of the objective and subjective problems surrounding deinstitutionalization is a necessary prerequisite to an after-care practice that insures the validity and provides the leadership to ex-patients in their struggle to integrate into the community as vital, dignified participants in daily life. In the following section of the book, we illustrate how this action orientation is used in diverse practice settings including case management programs, day treatment programs of various types, legal and legislative activities, program evaluation, and in community organizing and constituency building.

Section II

The Application of Problem Definition and Practice Principles to Different Arenas of Practice

Introduction

We turn now to detailed discussions of several different program areas that provide a context for the elucidation of the problem definition, practice principles and action orientation described in the first section of this book. We have selected the two most typical forms of practice in mental health after-care, case management and day programs, to demonstrate the viability of an advocacy/empowerment approach in direct practice with former psychiatric hospital patients. In addition, we have chosen to present the same problem definition approach and set of practice concerns in three other contexts – legal advocacy and organizing, program evaluation and community organization – because we believe these 'indirect' services are prerequisite to the implementation of an adequate, comprehensive, community-based mental health program.

Our direct practice chapters have a slightly different emphasis with regard to the working relationships involved in service delivery. We are assuming that the vast majority of case management work is done with individual clients and predominantly outside a professional office setting. In our case management chapter the focus is on work with individual clients who are presumed to be seen either in the 'homes' where they have been placed or at day programs to which they have been sent. Conversely, in our day program chapter, we are assuming that most work will be done with groups who meet in a designated program space outside the participants' residences. For this reason, in addition to discussion of the practice principles as applied to work with groups, we have presented material related to how our approach to practice is manifest in the physical appearance of a day program setting, in the organization of daily tasks and housekeeping responsibilities, etc.

The focus of direct practice is predominantly on the process of empowerment, of reconnecting the social, objective world to people's subjective experience in order to reflect critically on that world and change it. The purpose of our practice is to liberate people's capacity to produce socially meaningful activity from the confined realm of mental patient identity and the oppressive realm of daily life shaped by profit housing, lack of control over one's body and living situation, and the manipulations and mystifications inevitably embedded in psychiatric and psycho-social versions of reality. The practice chapters described will demonstrate principles directed toward transformation of both oppressive conditions and oppressive self-contempt which functions to reproduce the debasing environment of social life for most ex-patients. It will become clear that personal transformation and social action are seen as inextricable, mutually reinforcing dimensions to direct practice. These two dimensions also represent the two tendencies within our practice approach: advocacy, being more directed at the objective aspect of practice, empowerment being directed more at the process or development aspect with a greater attentiveness to the subjective dimension.

The chapters on legal advocacy and organizing, program evaluation, and community organization utilize the same framework for practice but emphasize the advocacy/objective dimension. Clearly, the scope of exploitation and oppression imposed upon ex-patients cannot be transformed through direct practice alone. These chapters inform after-care programs or workers on an array of activities that support the advocacy/empowerment orientation of the direct practice programs. The chapter on legal advocacy and organizing describes legal rights and entitlements materials and actions, and other legal and legislative strategies which lift issues of daily life out of the arena of daily direct practice interaction into broader and more overtly political forums. It also describes ways to promote sustained communication and development of interaction between direct practice components and the activities undertaken in the legal advocacy arena. Program evaluation, often seen by direct practice program staff as static, irrelevant and occasionally obligatory, is presented in the following chapter as an extension of direct practice concerns. It demonstrates how daily life issues for clients and staff can be critically assessed, how agenda setting for case management or day program staff and clients can be developed and how advocacy/empowerment-oriented programs can protect themselves from outside attack by more conventional service providers. The community organization chapter develops this theme and addresses the issue of constituency building for a community-based, alternatively construed program as well as addressing ways to promote greater and more positive interaction between ex-patients placed in community settings and their community's resources and residents.

CHAPTER 4

Case Management

Case managers, as one can quickly surmise from their title, are the invention of systems planners. Systems planners, in the human services field, are determined to locate problems within the existing boundaries of systems as they see them. The use of the title, 'Case Manager', suggests a wedding between conventional mental health clinicians comfortable with the term 'case' and systems planners comfortable with the use of 'manager.' These two influences permeate the suggested form of practice: case management emerges as a composite of a medical/psychiatric model for dealing with cases to be administered efficiently by managers accountable to a system. Taken together, this approach presumes and asserts a definition of the problems to be addressed which combines system maintenance with clinical reductionism, neither of which addresses the central problems faced by former mental patients residing in the community. On the surface, the typical tasks and functions required of case managers may seem quite benign, perhaps even helpful: who could object to working diligently to construct a comprehensive service plan, to coordinating a disparate array of service providers, to advocating for inaccessible services, etc.? But, just beneath the surface, there remains a far less rational yet systemic universe that constitutes the harsh social and economic reality of everyday life for most former patients. Sadly, this reality has little to do with the service model designed to be the panacea for hundreds of thousands of ex-patients by federal and state mental health planners.

In almost every model of case management, the major function of case managers is coordination of an array of services from numerous provider agencies in the community (Turner and TenHoor, 1978; Cox, 1981). Managing or constructing a coordinated service plan involving multiple social service and mental health agencies, from different jurisdictional levels (e.g., SSI/Medicaid/SRO housing), with different policies, guidelines and regulations has been problematic for people with far more institutional, organizational and political power than case managers. In fact, extensive research exists to demonstrate empirically that coordination and service integration efforts fare rather poorly (Rose, 1972; Warren *et al.*, 1974; Comptroller General, 1977), especially when new approaches to problems are proposed. It is indeed ironic that systems planners and administrators, having failed in their efforts at integrating and coordinating services, have now passed this responsibility on to those workers with the least power in the organizational structure, i.e., the 'line worker,' and have placed these responsibilities at the core of a new service delivery system. How case managers cope with these impossible coordination and integration tasks and functions is another story.

Political problems disguised as management problems

What makes the typical set of tasks given to case managers an impossible dream is that these responsibilities are operationally un-feasible and inherently contradictory. With little power to control their own agency's operations or concepts of problem definition, let alone the problem formulation practices or activities of other service provid-ers, case managers cannot demand or require either that their own agency or others produce appropriate services for their clients. This is especially true since coordination and interagency collaboration are achieved largely through voluntary or persuasion processes. A more realistic stimulant to the provision of community-based services for former patients has been the contracts provided by federal* or state mental health agencies. In addition, access to third party payments from Medicaid, allowing occasional dual payments, has brought a number of agencies into the mental health arena who previously had refused to offer services to former state hospital patients.

Where do all of these political and funding realities leave case managers? Most often, case managers, rather than creating or plan-

---

* Community Support Program funds from the National Institute of Mental Health.

ning a comprehensive system of care related to individual client's needs, are required to work out referrals and transportation to already existing services which have been designated as both appropriate and available because of contractual arrangements with funding and/or coordinating agencies. The real facilitating in case management is that related to reimbursement, since case managers are rarely offered the opportunity to be critical participants in program planning for their clients and rarely have the opportunity for critical input into needs definition, program design and/or evaluation of participating agencies. This statement does not imply that the need for such critical questioning ever occurs to most case managers. Clearly, it does not because the ideological paradigm of their own agency as well as that of other agencies does not allow the case manager to see him or herself as anything other than a deliverer of services in the traditional sense. Case management in most instances is reduced to connecting clients with various agencies whose track records for providing appropriate services for case management clients are non-existent or poor (Bachrach, 1976; Comptroller General, 1977; Turner and TenHoor, 1978).

The inevitable contradiction which befalls case managers therefore results from the dual expectation of combining coordination of services with advocacy. It is our belief that these two tasks – coordination and advocacy – cannot be assigned equal priority. Coordination, as a pre-eminent value, carries a set of assumptions with it about the various agencies that make up the ingredients of any comprehensive service plan. This assumption involves beliefs about the existence of a level of caring and about organizational flexibility. Such assumptions consciously or unconsciously place the existing service system in a position of primacy because the need for coordination presumes that those agencies whose services are being coordinated are aware of the real needs of clients (see Chapter 1) and are prepared to meet those needs. In reality, many agencies do what can be marketed for either contract dollars and/or reimbursement dollars; clients either 'fit' into the services offered by agencies and their service delivery models, or they do not receive the service. In this construction of reality, clients' needs are defined and confined to pre-existing services and patterns of organizational interaction with other agencies (Rose, 1972). When coordination is presented to case managers as their primary responsibility, advocacy-oriented activities are constrained by a priori commitments to those agencies or management strategies included in the coordinative planners' images and idealizations of service system integration. Advocacy, then, is shaped by the existing boundaries and practices of those agencies whose services are to be coordinated and advocacy efforts must stop short of producing harsh conflict with these agencies. Advocates operating within these parameters may demand that their clients have access to existing services, but they cannot make those services relevant to clients' needs or have them delivered in sensitive ways.

Advocacy, should it be given top priority, offers no a priori concessions as to the appropriateness of the services provided by existing agencies or programs. It asserts the primacy of clients' social needs as we have defined them in Chapter 1, and critically examines agencies and services in relation to their capacity to meet these needs in appropriate ways. Since our concept of advocacy is tied inextricably to empowerment, an agency's willingness to transfer power to clients, to engage them in planning and decision making about service utilization, and to make information as available to them as would be extended to other workers, all comprise the variables that determine potential interagency collaboration.

Advocating for appropriate services from this perspective most often produces harsh conflict in the inter-organizational arena of agencies supposedly involved in cooperative or coordinative service delivery agreements (Rose, 1972; Warren *et al.*, 1974). Thus, it appears that maintaining a commitment to coordination at the same time as one is committed to advocacy can occur only when the range of agencies involved agrees to common formulations of the problems to be addressed and to derived modalities of service (Kuhn, 1962): the nature of the agreement can either be modelled after conventional psychiatric or psycho-social problem definitions or from another framework, such as the advocacy/empowerment design we are proposing. Where the conventional psychiatric definitions prevail, coordination of services constitutes a betrayal of ex-patients as human beings, as a socially living person, for such a definition postulates the consumer-dependence of ex-patients upon services, landlords and agencies over which they have no control. It also functions to reconfirm mental patient identity as the clients' basis for relating to the social world.

Nowhere does this issue of problem definition manifest itself with the clarity that it does when we look at the typical housing situations of former psychiatric patients. For most people about to be discharged from state hospitals, housing options are narrow and are determined more by the availability of a bed than by the suitability of a particular environment to the individual's needs. Bed availability and the profit sector are intertwined in the area of deinstitutionalization as private entrepreneurs have developed a range of housing 'options' from Skilled Nursing Homes through Intermediate Care facilities to Adult Homes and SROs. Whatever the 'level of care' involved, the central force in all of these options is profit – extraction of private benefit from poor and relatively powerless people who serve as conduits to transfer public dollars (via SSI) to private ownership (Rose, 1972).

The profit motive of landlords and facility operators incorporates itself into the lives of ex-patients in insidious ways. For example, whenever even a small number of former patients reside in the same housing unit, it is typical to find the owner and/or manager of the building included on a 'treatment team,' involving also the hospital out-patient department or another mental health clinic, the County Social Services office, health or mental health service providers as well as case managers. The purpose of the 'team' is to coordinate and assure the delivery of medically modelled mental health and management services to residents of the home. Rarely is there perceived to be an overt conflict of interest involved between the not-for-profit service providers and the profit-motivated owners or managers whose income is dependent upon exploiting ex-patients. Joining this 'team' obviously compromises or eliminates a case manager's ability to do any advocacy work with clients centered around issues of tenants' rights or entitlements, access to more suitable services, criticism of existing services or service delivery patterns. Being a 'team' member also sets up clearly identifiable boundaries for clients with regard to sharing information about their life circumstances. Such a reaction is understandable since so many dimensions of clients' lives are frequently contoured by one or more of the agencies represented on the 'team.' In real terms, the 'team' constitutes a conspiracy of legitimated manipulation and self-interest. It upholds the validity of profit and legitimates its participating organizations while simultaneously invalidating clients by sustaining mental patient identities in community settings.

A similar situation occurs when case managers are invited to in-patient discharge planning conferences which are usually held in the hospital just prior to a patient's release. In these instances, workers representing the service agencies assumed by hospital staff to be 'appropriate' service providers are invited to participate in the preparation of what is considered to be a comprehensive service plan, a process which ostensibly also includes the patient. More realistically, the plan is prepared by whomever is assigned discharge planning responsibilities in the hospital (some hospitals have their own discharge planning departments, some members of whom plan without a thorough knowledge of the patient, while others have ward staff as planners) and includes all those agencies with whom the hospital has formal or informal working agreements. Usually this group includes only those agencies that have service contracts with the State Mental Health Department to operate after-care programs and the private profit homeowner/manager who has agreed to take the patient upon discharge. Often neglected in this procedure are the conflict of interest and violation of confidentiality involved in widespread sharing of information about one person without his or her informed consent. The participating case manager is placed in the position of agreeing to this process and ensuring that the terms of the plan are followed. Rarely does the patient object – to do so is grounds for being retained in the hospital. Should the case manager concur with the plan and/or the process and violation of confidentiality, especially in front of the patient, the case manager is immediately associated with the rest of the group ('team') whom the patient knows has the power to retain or return him/her to the hospital.

The world presumed to exist by policy-makers or by discharge planners and the reality lived by former patients differ from one another in significant ways. The ex-patient, particularly, if she/he has been in and out of the hospital previously, knows what the contours of daily life will be: inadequate, unsafe or poorly run profit housing dominated by management (in licensed places) and/or by violence (SROs); poverty; medication-addicted psychiatrists (see Scull, 1977, chapter on 'The Technological Fix'); monotonous, repetitive, infantalizing day programs or workshops (see Chapter 5); and inadequate health care. The discharge plan conceals the truth of this reality as thoroughly as it validates the existing service delivery system and its approach to clients' needs. Case managers participating in activities that disguise conflicts of interest in the guise of a 'team' are in danger of being coopted into the concealed or mystified reality that is so important to the maintenance of the agency system. For a case manager to cooperate and coordinate within the confines of such a system of 'care' means that, for his or her clients, the contours of daily life can never be other than those described above. Such a way of working, therefore, constitutes collusion, however inadvertent, on the part of the case manager in a service delivery system which allows for the continued manipulation, domination and exploitation of clients.

It is not necessary for a case manager to participate acquiescently in such a manipulative and mystifying ritual. Case managers can initiate contact with clients or potential clients at discharge planning sessions by adhering to the intent of discharge planning which is to involve patients in planning for their release. The case manager can ask about the patient's involvement in the discharge planning process: Has she/he been to visit the housing option selected for her/him? Were other places explored and visited? What were the criteria used to choose the housing selected? How did the hospital staff determine the level of care required? Did the patient agree with the choice of criteria and the level of care? Did the patient understand the purpose of the discharge planning meeting? What was her/his understanding of the role of the other participants in the meeting? Did the patient have the opportunity to talk to peers about what it is like to live in the place selected for housing or to take part in the services offered by the providers attending the discharge meeting?

These questions are suggestive of our approach to case management services. In the remainder of this chapter, we will try to articulate how the theory presented in the first section of this book is operationalized in our case management practice.

A stereotypic view of the life of a former state psychiatric hospital patient is presented rather simply: all the needs of the clients are taken care of by service providers, leaving the former patient with few concerns related to day-to-day survival (the only exception being 'bag ladies' and other chronically resistant types). Because all of their needs are being attended to, former patients have little to do but sit around all day watching television or attending day programs designed for them. The truth, of course, is starkly different: regardless of an individual's particular social, medical and/or psychological circumstances, the reality of daily life for most ex-patients is, at best, difficult and, at worst, very harsh. Problems with income, housing and health care are constants in the lives of most former patients. To respond to these problems requires an extensive working knowledge of a remarkable array of agencies and service bureaucracies from a multitude of political jurisdictions including federal, state and local governments, voluntary sector service providers, courts, regulatory agencies and local organizations. These institutions are omnipresent in the life of

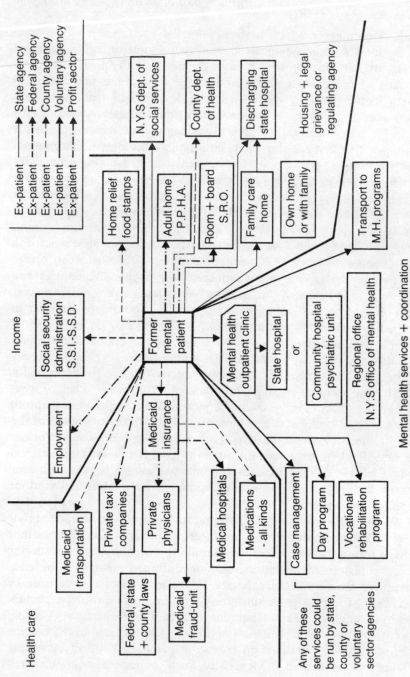

Figure 4.1 A common multi-jurisdictional picture of the inter-organizational environment of the ex-mental patient

former patients as we illustrate in Figure 4.1.

Figure 4.1 is an attempt to show how the inter-organizational and inter-jurisdictional areas can shape former patients' lives. The complexity of an existence where all areas of concrete or real needs are controlled by others, coupled with the docile, 'adaptive' mental patient identity, creates a situation similar to hospital life where passive acquiescence is adopted in order to get minimal survival needs met. It is imperative that case managers understand this inter-organizational system and its impact upon former patients' lives. This process involves understanding that every agency has its own set of policies, guidelines and regulations for each program it offers; that each has its own formal and informal administrative structure and operational processes; that each has its own individual workers who understand their jobs in a certain way; and that each person in each agency acts as a 'gatekeeper' or overseer of needed resources. Obviously, the former patient perceives everyone connected with such bureaucracies and agencies as obstacles or threats to be overcome. In each case, agencies can be expected to fight to maintain their own boundaries, their own expedient means of operating, their own ways of defining clients' problems and delivering services, and their perception of their own validity and viability. While workers within each agency will certainly vary to some degree, they all can be expected to know primarily about their own agency and substantially less about every other agency. When the focus turns to clients' concrete, real, social needs, and to clients' legal rights and entitlements, most workers involved in the mental health after-care system know very little. The scant information available to them usually concerns legal rights and entitlements, which benefit their agency or the homeowner as well as the client, for example, procedures necessary for obtaining a Medicaid card or application procedures for SSI.

We view the case manager's central responsibility to be understanding both the complex network of inter-organizational operations that shape former patients' lives, and seeing this system in relation to our clients' history of powerlessness and enforced passivity. The case manager must have the capacity to see most clients as capable of struggling to gain greater autonomy, of becoming more active participants in determining what happens to them. But the necessary starting point, we believe, for such an approach is knowledge of the service delivery system, understood from the perspective of advocacy for rights and entitlements. Minimally, such an understanding involves knowing the functions and responsibilities for your own agency and for every other agency in the inter-organizational network; knowing where power and decision-making authority are located (e.g., who decides what issue); understanding how informal systems work; and how any formal grievance mechanisms (such as fair hearings) operate. We see the development of this information and the teaching of it to staff to be major tasks for any agency committed to an advocacy/empowerment design. We will make some suggestions about how these responsibilities can be pursued in Chapter 6.

We assume our practice with any client must begin with the case manager's assessment of that person's capacity to describe the life she/he lives and to translate what are presented as complaints into issues able to be acted upon. In addition, a case manager must attempt to learn what the client already knows about his or her rights and entitlements, particularly those rights and entitlements most applicable to the complaints voiced by the client. Equally important, the case manager must attempt to learn how each client thinks and feels about him/herself and his/her living situation. Thus, our practice with any client will emerge from the individual client's present level of knowledge about the systems which impact on his/her life and from his/her self-concept as expressed in behavior towards us, in self-perception and in his/her scope of information about basic needs. We then move from this point to a process of continuing elaboration and assessment with the client of the immediate forces and structures impinging upon his or her everyday life.

Having information about legal rights and entitlements readily at hand, or knowing how and where to get it, provides the case manager with immediate resources to share with former patients. Introducing legal rights and entitlements information into a discussion with clients suggests a different approach than that of other agencies. To further emphasize this difference, we suggest using a client-resource check list early in the preliminary phase of client contact. Our check list identifies concrete issues, problems and resources devoid of medical model problem definitions. The list is used as a way of simultaneously introducing the new worker (case manager) and a new perspective to clients. Here are some of the materials we have used:

Case Management, Client Check List

1   Our agency's Community Support Systems Information packet.

    Describes case management program and day program, with names, addresses and telephone numbers included along with meeting times for day program.

2   Eligibility Form – a State Office of Mental Health form that we are required to fill out (copy given to client).

3   Office of Mental Health consent form, releasing state hospital to give dates of hospitalization to Community Support Systems agencies. Necessary for eligibility (copy given to client with information about our interpretation of confidentiality).

4   Information about how to get and use Medicaid transportation.

5   Bus routes along a map of the area.

6   Handicapped ID form and information packet (for use in getting reduced bus fares and for general identification purposes).

7   Adult Home or SRO legal rights/entitlements booklet (copy given to client).

8   Voter registration packet (given to client).

9   Rent rebate – State Income Tax Rebate form (copy given to client).

The list refers to several forms that agencies often use to determine client eligibility for case management services, forms which many clients have never seen. We openly share and explain these forms to clients. Our check list also contains such information as specifics about public transportation, information meant to introduce discussion about the client's knowledge of the geographical setting, and to communicate to the person that we do not see him/her as bound by the mental health transportation system (if there is one) which only takes people to legitimated mental health programs. Other information is included that introduces the client to the local world of community life, not as a mental patient, but as a citizen, all of which communicates who we are and provides a beginning point for our approach to redefining problems and sharing a process outside the medical-psychiatric model.

Quite obviously, we are not recommending that a case manager simply introduce him/herself and commence reading a litany of legal rights and entitlements. Rather, we are suggesting that the first contacts with clients must express some substantive difference from the medicalized and/or 'service coordination' orientation of other service providers. This difference must also be reflected in the *process* of interactions, perhaps through honest commentary on the situation at hand, or in refusing to sign a discharge plan in which the patient has not actively participated or in acknowledging that the case manager is not part of any 'treatment team.' In any case, we believe that first contacts are the time to tell the client briefly about the case manager's commitment to exploring the client's interests in available services, legal rights and benefits, etc.

Our advocacy/empowerment orientation requires that communication with clients be directed toward engaging them in critical discussion about the conditions of their daily lives. Such discussion may include an exploration of the causes of these conditions, the client's thoughts and feelings concerning his/her situation, and the relationship between the client's perceptions of what he/she needs and available services. We do not present ourselves as legalistic, that is, interested in the client only as he/she reflects a legal issue of concern to us, or as interested only in service delivery to the exclusion of trying to know the client as an individual. Rather, we want to stake out our turf: we see the client as a socially human being, living in conditions which are socially and historically understandable and which are at least somewhat permeable. We also communicate to clients that our commitment is to build a client-case manager relationship centered around a commitment for change. We want each client to know that we do not accept his or her mental patient identity as a fixed, impermeable statement about who he or she is. At the same time, we do acknowledge the existence of this identity as a starting point for our work together.

We assume that most clients initially will present themselves to us through their learned, socially constructed mental patient identities and designated social roles. In part, this way of presenting themselves reflects the mental patient-like environments found in most community placements, replicating the worst aspects of institutional care and thus demanding that ex-patients' behavior and self-concept remain institutionalized. In part, mental patient identity also reflects the experience people have had with mental health and/or social services workers whose own identities and roles form the counterpart to mental patienthood.

While there certainly are some variations in behavior and presentation of self within socially defined 'mental patient' identity, common patterns are clearly recognizable: a generally obsequious manner, a posture communicating an incorporated invalidation, and/or a frequently expressed acquiescence to anticipated demands or expectations, etc. Often these behaviors mask feelings of inferiority, of failure and incompetence, of a generalized self-contempt. Behaviourally, the feelings are also demonstrated through commonly recurring complaints about being tired, having a headache, having to go to his or her room to lie down, having to ask others to do even simple things for them (unless there is an instant reward of food or money). When invited to participate in activities such as described in Chapter 5, people often initially respond that they are too tired, afraid to go out, etc. In some younger ex-patients, beneficiaries of the modern era of mental health treatment, many similar characteristics are demonstrated: a fear or threat that their symptoms will reappear, a reification of their 'sickness' and terror of its omnipresent nature, all of which are harbingers of a return once again to the hospital. In other younger patients, an ironic reversal of these postures is expressed through an obviously false, exaggerated self-assurance (particularly among males), pseudo-independence, declarations about having no need for services, particularly those related to their frequently deplorable housing situations. Any negatives found in current conditions are presented to workers as largely irrelevant because these housing arrangements are only temporary way stations being used until the younger ex-patients get themselves back on their feet.

Whether the expression of mental patient identity shows itself in the form of a person who appears fragile, permanently impaired and predominantly dependent or in the form of a hardened, pseudo-autonomous appearing individual, we must understand the influence of imposed mental patient identity on all communication between former patients and mental health workers, particularly in the early phases of contact. Ex-patients must be expected either to be wary or cynical about meeting workers who arrive to tell them about new types of services or programs available to them. It is exactly for this reason that we attempt to pose problems to clients' inevitable set of justified expectations about service providers (agency workers). The problem-posing approach we take is both substantive and process-oriented. It is substantive in relation to the issues presented to clients upon first contact (see client check list on pp. 83–4) and with regard to our adamant stand on confidentiality. It is process-orientated in our interaction with clients, an interaction which includes sharing of information, a commitment to letting the client control the choice of which, if any, services she/he will use, and to identify the issues which will be the focus of client-case management interactions. This way of presenting ourselves, with substantive issues coupled to process commitments which are mutually reinforcing, constitutes a type of confrontation to mental patient identity and role behavior. It is our hope and expectation that the challenge posed by our practice will act as an invitation to the person to reflect critically on his/her situation with the purpose of changing the oppressive conditions of his/her daily life rather than acting to reproduce them.

Central to this problem-posing approach to practice is the development of dialogue with clients, a process of communication quite different from interviewing skills or other method-based psychotherapeutic encounters. Dialogue assumes that the person involved has a view of the world and of him/herself in it, however incorrect, distorted, or disguised that view may be. Dialogue presumes that with encouragement and validation of the right to think and feel as a person (beyond the contours of mental patient identity), people will share their perceptions and experience. A commitment to dialogue involves a continuous support for clients to allow them to elaborate on what they perceive to be happening to them and around them. Such elaboration will also include descriptions of what they are feeling about themselves and their situations, and an accounting of why they think things are organized as they are. The issue of who benefits from current conditions becomes, over time, a natural question to be raised.

Our case managers work towards connecting subjective experience (perception and feelings) to objective conditions (the social base of poverty, landlord-tenant relations, doctor-patient relationships etc.). The commitment to engage people in dialogue requires that clients participate in the analysis of the problems confronting them as well as in the deliberation of possible action strategies. This requirement to involve ex-patients in examining their own life situations and acting to produce chosen outcomes presents an ongoing dilemma for case managers: it is often far easier to do things *for* clients rather than to engage them in dialogue and mutual strategy development. Moreover, the problem-solving direction inherent in the 'doing for' approach to case management is more comfortable to most workers, more contiguous with their own life situations, more certain and rewarding. Initially, it is also more compatible with mental patient identity and, therefore, appears to produce more positive feedback. Involvement, development and mutual participation of clients is uncertain, demanding more trust in clients as people, rather than in trusting mental patient identity, bureaucratic negotiations, stratified power relations, existing power relationships and continued dependency.

Problem-solving as opposed to problem-posing most often functions to obscure and obstruct clients' understanding of the deeper reasons (causes) behind the problems they face: it suggests a relatively facile process of advocacy and change, augmented by the knowledge and skill of the expert worker, thus communicating to clients that their passive manner produces desired outcomes. Problem-solving can usurp or pre-empt a client's right to develop the capacity to function more independently as a person living in the community, or to gain some measure of control over aspects of daily life. While our case managers certainly do not sit passively, for example, when people are threatened with eviction or with SSI decertification, we are reluctant to 'solve' the problem presented unless a crisis situation is in progress. Even in situations requiring immediate action, unless they are life threatening, we struggle to have the client know exactly what is going on, to know why the situation at hand exists as it does, and to determine his/her choice of action. An atypical example of this might be a crisis situation in which the homeowner or manager, along with other mental health agency workers from the 'team,' are trying to convince an ex-patient to return voluntarily to the hospital. Our role would involve trying to talk to the person-in-crisis, trying to learn how much choice and knowledge is experienced in the moment (if any), and to seek alternatives, where possible (e.g., a temporary crisis residence). Owners or managers and 'team' members will oppose this intervention, requiring that the worker have a ready source of support (other staff members) available either to come directly to the situation or to offer counsel by telephone.

Our view of practice requires that after resolving a problem, or even failing to resolve one, the process must be explored: who defined the problem? How did the problem get defined in that way? How did the client feel about her/his participation in what took place? What has the client learned from the interaction? What has the case manager learned? These are questions for mutual exploration and are necessary for identifying or posing problems yet to be confronted.

The central direct practice task for case managers is to stimulate dialogue directed toward critical reflection with people about their perceptions of the reality of their daily life experiences. We seek to elicit people's perceptions of their situations, to help them identify where these perceptions come from, and to create with them an elaboration of their thoughts and feelings about themselves as socially alive persons struggling to live as social historical beings (people) rather than to exist simply as mental patients 'displaced' into communities. The intention of this type of communication is the repeated effort to reconnect subjectivity with objectivity, to re-establish communication between objective conditions (e.g., powerlessness, the oppression of poverty or stigma, etc.) and an individual's feelings about her or himself in the context in which she or he lives. This capacity for dialectical appraisal (the continuous objective/subjective relation) is pivotal in our concept of personal development.

We emphasize the relation of objective conditions and subjective experience in all discussions with clients. For example, when a client raises a complaint about her or his residence, a case manager, through the process of elaboration, will attempt to learn the scope of the client's criticism, the client's perception about what can be done, and the client's perception of him/herself as a producer of change. Along the way, the case manager also will inquire about the client's feelings as reflections of his/her thoughts about his/her situation and him/herself as a potentially active participant in determining the outcome. Interaction initiated in those ways is followed up by raising critical questions about the commonplace; for example, why does the homeowner hold a client's Medicaid card? Has the client seen the face of his/her monthly cheque, and what figure is written there? Where does the Medicaid card or SSI cheque come from? Are there rules or regulations about these issues or other questions related to housing?

Case managers are struggling in every way to communicate to our clients that they are social beings, living in a particular context that can be known and eventually acted upon in a way which furthers their own interests: that their lives can be something more than a facile conduit for third party payments to landlords and social agencies. Movement in this struggle can only advance when ex-patients are able to contemplate themselves as people experiencing objectifiably knowable circumstances. These circumstances are then perceptually transformed from the 'natural' or 'inevitable' to socially acknowledged historical facts. As they were humanly created and maintained, so can they be acted upon by people and changed over time. Knowledge is produced in this process rather than simply transferred or consumed by workers or clients.

When oppressed people can come to recognize some aspect of the nature of their oppression – perhaps its historicity or its social function – some alteration occurs in their self-concept. If one sees oneself as devalued in an ahistorical manner, for example, as a biological defect or medical object, one's capacity to comprehend the social nature of oppression and one's place within it is mystified, distorted and obstructed. As one comes to understand the social existence of the oppressive contours of daily life, the potential for change, for producing daily life in some different form, becomes plausible. It is only in this context, of perceiving oneself somehow able to struggle to produce change, that there exists a challenge and an opportunity to transform the self-contempt which the oppressors have forced mental patients to internalize and which maintains itself through daily behavior patterns. Therefore, the struggle to transform the imposed social identity of mental patient requires that it be externalized or understood as a social construction which serves the interests of various groups of people while being antagonistic to the people upon whom it is imposed. This assumption then frames a significant part of our practice strategy: staff work with people to elaborate their perceptions of existing circumstances, help clients to reflect critically about the causes of these life circumstances, and encourage clients to reflect about how and why they see and feel about themselves as they do. This process will be guided toward some client-determined change effort, using an interim strategy we refer to as limit-situations (from Freire, see Chapter 3 of *Pedagogy of the Oppressed*, 1968).

Any action directed toward change in the objective context externalizes problems, redefines problems as being contextual, and thus opens possibilities for exploration of subjective transformation as well. For this reason we work very hard to have people engaging in change efforts of any type or level talk them through, whether in case management or at a day program. The purpose of elaborating *the experience of the process* as it develops is to allow people to perceive themselves changing through their own self-selected and self-directed actions, through seizing command of some aspect (however minute) of their daily lives. In so doing, *the people are externalizing the basis for the self-contempt that has been built into their identities over the years and re-internalizing an opposing positive self-perception. As people speak out loud about themselves, understanding their social world and acting to change it, they are simultaneously transforming the concept they hold of themselves as incapable of either social comprehension or positive action.* Therefore, at the center of the process of elaboration is the confrontation between being a passive consumer, known and acted upon, and becoming an active participant who learns to know and act. Social action in accord with one's defined interests and social transformation of one's self-concept or identity-in-the-world thus emerge as mutually required dimensions of our practice. Either aspect can become a focal point so long as the connection between them is clearly understood and pursued.

Since the basis for identity comes from historical social experience together with current contextual social life, either dimension can become a starting point for the process of change. We have focused more directly on beginning change efforts with the objective conditions of daily life because we believe that we can engage people more successfully at this level: the issues are readily at hand, people have multiple complaints about living conditions (see material below about complaining as the only available form of mental patient criticism), and materials are immediately available (e.g., rights and entitlements laws and regulations) to use as a response which poses the types of problems we have been describing. It is also the case that ex-patients have had so much exposure to everything resembling therapy (subjectivism) that efforts at responding to the subjective dimension initially seem to produce a very healthy 'resistance' or well-developed game-playing posture (the functional acquiescence mentioned earlier).

The descriptions of the processes of elaboration and dialogue which we have just detailed are meant to be viewed as guides, processes to be developed over time, ensuring that the central focus of our case management relationship is not lost. The relationship between clients and case managers evolves and is built upon trust, validation and support for the client as a human being expressing his/her past history and present identity. At the risk of being repetitive, we again want to assert our premise that when the client is understood to be a social historical person, it is very different from the client who is seen as a 'mental patient.' The difference in perception represents a critical reflection on what happens to a person in our mental health system. Case management, from our perspective, has the task of working to develop the client/person's capacity to participate consciously in his/her life and, in so doing, to reinforce his/her valid human experience and activity. This, in turn, will act back on the person's concept of identity: invalid, mental patient activity reproduces invalid, mental patient identity as systematically as valid social activity challenges that negative identity and poses an alternative to it. Following this premise, quite obviously we are required to reflect on interaction patterns between our clients and mental health professionals, as well as on the substance of these interactions. This reflection is necessary because the identity assumed by the former patient is a reflection of the social roles and identity held by their previous caretakers. Put another way, there is a consistency between the substance and process of communication used by professionals. who operate out of a psychiatric paradigm and the passive, acquiescent, devalued mental patient role behaviour observed in clients. We must challenge both the substance of that interaction pattern and the process. Our orientation, which requires that attention be directed toward the concrete world of everyday life as discussed at length above, and illustrated by Figure 4.1 and the client check list, represents much of the substance of our view. But more must be done to counter clients' experiences derived from what may be many years of typical interaction with mental health programs guided by the psychiatric world view.

One vehicle for posing a problem to conventional relationships with 'helpers' is grounded in our position on confidentiality. For most clients, to the extent that they have heard of confidentiality, the definition of its meaning has come from within mental health practice or policy. Generally, this interpretation in practice has meant that the mental health professional could share whatever information with whomever she/he chose, with the operational ethic being expedience. Our experience has been that professional and paraprofessional workers routinely violate confidentiality by talking without a client's specific consent to professionals from other agencies and to homeowners or managers considered to be part of a formal or informal 'treatment team.' Clients generally know this process happens because it is not unusual for violations of confidentiality to occur in front of them, all done in the name of caretaking and coordination and presumed to be necessary to the effective delivery of services.

We define confidentiality differently: we will communicate absolutely nothing about a client to anyone else, under any circumstances short of life threatening situations, unless authorized explicitly by the person in writing to do so. Further, we interpret *informed* consent to mean that the client must know what information is being authorized to be shared with whom and for what reason. Without this level of informed participation, we will neither send information to other agencies, nor honor their requests for such information, an act which has produced considerable conflict for us. We have found that other agencies commonly have blank consent forms which clients are told to sign in advance, with neither specific purposes nor a specified time period listed. We will not respond to these forms without first checking with the client to make sure she/he knows what is being requested and for what reasons. The fact that we will not compromise on this issue, even in the face of threats and harassment from other agencies, has helped to build trust with a number of clients. Such action has also communicated to people that our concept of practice is rooted more firmly in their human dignity and its legal guarantees than in typical mental health agency practice or policy.

Over time, trust with clients is further developed as they observe the marked difference between our relationships with home-owners and those of other service providers. From our first contact with a client, when we may present him or her with the check list or legal rights booklets, our view of the person is clearly conveyed: we see clients as rent-paying tenants, legally entitled to be treated as such; and we view clients' comments and complaints about their life circumstances as valid and serious criticisms of their objective reality. Further, we see homeowners and/or managers as profiteers, not as caretakers or 'team members.'

The struggle of our practice approach is to transform complaints into serious, legitimate critical commentary about living conditions. We pursue this process by beginning to produce an elaboration directed toward what the client sees as the problem or the basis for complaining (however superficial, exaggerated or irrelevant the complaint may seem to us at times); about how the problem came into being; about why the problem exists as it does; about who is involved in the situation and what the role of each person is; about what the problem creates in terms of the client's feelings about him/herself and the situation; about what possible actions might be taken; and about what projected repercussions might come from each projected action. This process is attempted whether the problem is one that is as immediately urgent as a decertification letter from SSI or one that is of a more ongoing nature such as a complaint about the quantity and/or quality of the food in an SRO. Whatever the issue, the process of trying to develop a more elaborate picture remains the same. And we struggle to do this process of elaboration even with people whose present circumstances or personal condition have created ways of expressing themselves which we cannot understand or to which we cannot relate, for example, people who are acting 'crazy' and remain aloof from the social world in which decisions about them are being made by others. In these instances, we quietly try to inform the person about what is going on, about our inability to communicate with her/him at present, and about our interest in returning when another type of interaction might be possible.

When people are assumed to be legitimate commentators about their social situation, they, too, have to take their situation more seriously. Workers are taught to represent to clients what they have heard from them, but filtered through the case manager's critical consciousness. This representation is most often done by introducing into the discussions information about violations of legal rights or about the existence of entitlements (a tax rebate issue has served as a good example because it can be income producing and therefore immediately attracts attention, even of people who previously were reluctant to work with us – see Appendix I). Our case managers take what clients have presented, struggle with them to build an elaboration of the issue and represent the information to clients. All of this acts as part of a process of validation of people's right to be treated as serious adults. The process also serves as recognition of their capacity to become critics/participants/actors on issues which concern their lives.

As case managers learn more from clients, the workers gain greater insight into clients' experience/perception of daily life. As this process occurs, two opportunities arise: to bring clients together to discuss common expressed concerns (only, however, with each person's permission to mention getting together with others, if they cannot do the organizing themselves); and the introduction of what Freire calls 'thematization'. This latter ingredient introduces concealed or mystified political content into the dialogue (e.g., differentiating a private profiteer from 'helpers' or 'caretakers'). Clients working through issues and exploring thematic content together not only strengthens the position taken on any issue, but further develops the relation between objective conditions and subjectivity. This objective/subjective connection is made through dialogue shared by people whose lives have much in common and who can collectively reflect on the feelings and perceptions flowing from their common base of shared circumstances rather than enduring them and reproducing themselves in isolation from one another.

As Freire noted, people who have been oppressed present their perceptions of themselves and their lives filtered through prevailing ideology and particular beliefs that often incorporate what their oppressors have thought of them. This ironic contradiction, in which one's self-contempt gives credence and legitimacy to one's oppressors, is a common 'hidden injury' (Sennett and Cobb, 1973) among oppressed people. Legitimizing the views of one's oppressors functions to conceal powerlessness and to legitimate authority. In the case of former mental patients, accepting as real the motion of 'mental patient' with all of the self-contempt and worthlessness contained in that view, also distorts much of the dismal reality that ex-patients share in common in the form of inadequate housing and income, poor health care, and lack of meaningful social activity. The inference is that former patients are getting what they deserve in the form of difficult life circumstances. Moreover, the elements which characterize the harsh living conditions and experience of daily life for former patients comprise the components of a 'treatment plan' and are presented as 'care' or 'service delivery.' Defining objective reality in this way not only precludes any critical questioning of what is received, but also serves to mystify the domination, exploitation and manipulation that occur. Demystification of objective reality is the purpose of thematization.

Giving respectability to one's oppressors simultaneously devalues the self and one's capability in identifying either the concrete problems of daily life or their causes. Consequently, when our case managers do hear criticisms, they come concealed, or in disguises, for example, as passive complaints or whining, so common to groups of people who perceive themselves (correctly) to be substantially powerless, while attributing legitimacy to those more powerful. What is being communicated in these instances is a criticism which appears to have no legitimate basis, either in the critic him/herself or in objective reality. All concealed forms of criticism are seriously pursued, both to give legitimation to the critic and validation to the commentary. At the same time, we realize that the plethora of complaints about the landlord, the staff, the food, the filth, the clinic, the medication, etc., carries with it an implied level of generality that transcends the very specific descriptive content of whatever any particular complaint may be. This level of generality is the thematic level of understanding, that is, what is being presented descriptively and passively is a hidden form of reaction to being powerless, delegitimated and dominated.

Because these latter thematic reflections of social reality derive from a framework of critical analysis which is unfamiliar, that is, from an analysis which acknowledges the existence of powerlessness, domination and exploitation as common elements in the lives of oppressed peoples, people experience the existence of these themes in disguised forms. These forms often appear as unidentifiable anger, obsequious complaining and/or feelings of inadequacy or incompetence. When the content inherent in these themes is experienced emotionally, without

an immediate conceptual framework available to make them understandable, both the concepts and the people who experience them in a
concealed form are denigrated. Feelings of delegitimacy occur because
people who do not have an ideologically clear or immediately available, legitimated frame of reference which conceptualizes their feelings in a logical world view react with intense fear and often assume
they are 'crazy.' For ex-patients, the fear is focused on the terror of
recurring symptoms, of being seen as 'decompensating' and of being
returned to the hospital.

It is our task to help make the thematic content of people's lives clear
to them through the process of dialogue. Case managers, through the
use of critical reflection, can help produce political clarity about social
reality by elevating the elaborated descriptive material elicited from
clients to a thematic level. A case manager's capacity for critical
reflection derives from an acknowledgment of the themes of oppression, domination and exploitation in our society, and an understanding
of how these themes are reflected in the lives of former patients. Such
an understanding allows the case manager to redefine the problems
faced by the ex-patient (see Chapter 1), identifies the thematic content, and allows the objective base of the problems to be unveiled. In
representing these themes to clients, former patients can come to see
common thematic threads recurrent in their lives.

The process of long-range case management constitutes an exploration of daily life as it presently exists and moves to a critical examination of why it is that way. It is made possible by descriptive elaboration
of perceptions and feelings by thematization, representation and
dialogue, all of which establish the preconditions for action. This is
based upon what we refer to as 'recontextualization' or the reconnection of the person to his/her social historical context as an active
participant. In the process, a reformulation of needs and problems
develops as the basis for possible action strategies and reformulation of
the actors' identities.

While contemplating potential actions, a second form of thematization occurs. Initially, as discussed above, we anticipate that people will
be docile/passive/adaptive to imposed dictates about reality. This
incorporation of a closed system or, as Freire calls it, a 'circle of
certainty,' is inherent in mental patient identity and is an essential
element in its internal collaboration with the sources of social control.
This 'circle of certainty' expresses itself in the life of the former patient
as an acceptance of his or her situation as it is, as impermeable and

incapable of being changed. Into this fixed view of the world, experience is introduced by case managers which continuously contradicts existing beliefs, for example, rights and entitlements data or a non-condescending way of talking to people which exemplifies another use of thematization. Here the themes involved are directly focused on people's fixed view of the world; on the meaning of this fixed view in terms of self-concept; and on exploration of who benefits from such perceptions. Presenting ideas about how to relate to new information, for example, about legal rights, entitlements or advocacy consists of representing perceptions clients have shared which are focused on single problem areas rather than on the totality of the problem situation. The larger critical analytic framework, discussed in Chapter 1, becomes the backdrop for framing more specific and limited problem formats. For example, struggling to identify a way to get a client's personal allowance (SSI) from an adult home landlord includes a problem-posing elaboration of landlord-tenant relations which encompasses, but is not synonomous with, the money issue. Problems are defined as identifiable limit situations in order to create possibilities for action in the otherwise stagnant and static-appearing social world of most ex-patients.

Once clients can begin to contemplate taking some form of action to represent their interests, a major breakthrough has occurred. This breakthrough on the part of the former patient represents tremendous change no matter how major or minor the particular issue may be. Contemplating action reflects a change from seeing the world and one's position in it as permanent and fixed to seeing it as permeable, as capable of being changed; it reflects movement from a position of consumer of an imposed reality to a position of partial producer of one's reality; and it reflects movement from a position of passive receiver of the dictates of others to a position of strategic responder to power relations. Put another way, contemplating action to change one's reality reflects movement from a caste-orientation to one of class status. All of these latter shifts occur at levels of thematic abstraction and may not, at first, be noticeable or perceived. These changes can be seen, nonetheless, in initially small alterations in a client's self-concept and way of relating to case managers or homeowners. In relation to case management, indicators of such change might be an increase in the quantity and/or quality of client-initiated issues for discussion, increased preparation by a client in anticipation of deliberation on an issue, etc. In relation to homeowners, the change might show itself in a specific refusal to be cowed, a demand to have a box lunch prepared, a willingness to discuss the existence of an 'informer' among day program participants, etc.

As we introduce probes about potential action, and reflect back on the situations described to us, we are using thematization to pose problems to the clients which are amenable to intervention by them. The process of eventual decision making about the mode and most appropriate strategy of intervention is preceded by reformulating a definition of the problem which makes it amenable to intervention. In addition, all possible action strategies are explored within the framework of evaluating benefits to be gained in relation to the risks taken for each potential strategic act. At this point, the process moves from the point of thematizing to what we call problematizing: the redefinition of a totality of impermeable oppression into a partialized or limited area where action can be contemplated and critically evaluated. During problematization, tactics can be discussed and decided on for moving ahead or a decision can be made, for strategic reasons, to take no action.

The following is an example of a time when clients might decide to refrain from action. A group of clients, learning about the benefits involved in SSI, come to discover that their landlord is illegally taking personal allowance money from them each month. They learn that there exists a body of law which protects them from this injury and that there are legal services lawyers who will represent them without fee, as well as regulatory agencies who are supposed to protect them. They explore the possible avenues for asserting their rights against their landlord, but ultimately decide to refrain from action because they are afraid of their landlord's power to return them to the hospital for 'acting out.' The choice, in this case, not to act on available options, is a strategic choice based on a critical evaluation of the benefits and risks and is not a reproduction of passive 'mental patient' acquiescence. It is an informed decision made possible through the case manager's work with clients to redefine the problem, partialize it, explore all possible avenues of action and weigh the benefits and risks of each. In this case, even the decision not to act against the power of the homeowner strengthens the ex-patients' capacity to see oppression, reflect on it critically, and build a stronger base for later action.

Because so many aspects of clients' lives are controlled by others, even to the extent of homeowners/landlords 'teaming up' with mental health professionals, we must be vigilant in order to ensure that clients' decisions to take action or not to take action on any given issue reflect their own decision making. We must beware of subtly coercing clients to act in ways that satisfy our needs as workers, but are not necessarily in the clients' best interests. At times, particularly when the causes of oppression appear self-evident to us and the injuries to people seem severe, the choice not to act can produce a strong negative reaction from case managers. In the example given above, we must guard against making judgments condemning the people for their failure to act as we might have wanted them to do, especially when the issue is one of heightened value to us. At these times, we must remember the life circumstances of the people contemplating action. We must remember that they are being asked to act against others with overwhelming power in their lives; and we must remember what the risks are to the clients. It is useful for case managers to recall the fear that former patients must feel when asked to contemplate acting outside the boundaries set for them and to remember that one result of any action on the part of an ex-patient may be rehospitalization.

We cannot overemphasize the principle that there can never be an issue which is more important than the lives of the people from which that issue arises, that the value of the people transcends the value of the issue at all times. To ignore this principle is to manipulate the clients, to transform them into our possessions, just as the traditional service providers presume formerly institutionalized clients to be the possessions of private proprietary homeowners or of the mental health system. To act toward people as if they were our objects to be manipulated as we choose constitutes betrayal. However, there are times when we, too, get caught up in the momentum or intensity of an issue and lose sight of the fact that the risks from any action are unequally distributed. We sometimes forget that the client most often has far, far more to lose than the worker(s) involved. This issue of client manipulation has come up even in our work with other agencies having similar practice commitments. For example, in our collaborative efforts with public interest lawyers, whose services are immensely valuable to our clients and to whom we refer regularly, we have sometimes found ourselves playing a recurring role wherein we must reinforce the fact that the client is the center of attention and the locus for all informed decision making. In this way, even legal actions become process or development-oriented, rather than short term, win/lose events. Within this framework, whatever the outcome of an event, it can be reflected upon for deeper critical understanding. The issue can then have 'empowerment' value even when it does not develop into a more aggressive action strategy.

Our approach to case management will not work with every client. There will be people with advanced organic brain disease who will be inappropriately placed in the facilities where we offer services and for whom we will have to assume a more directive role to assure that adequate services are delivered. There will be people whose level of fear will prevent even the thought of challenging authority (landlords or managers, for example) and they will refuse to work with us. Moreover, there will be people who will find our problem-posing process too threatening to participate in, regardless of the fact they are never pushed to move in a direction they do not want for themselves. In all of these instances, and many others which arise, our position is the same: we continue to present ourselves in the same way; we continue to attempt to engage people at whatever level we can reach them, on whatever topic is of interest to them; and we continue to present our concerns about their social existence. We also inform clients who decline our services, or who decide to withdraw from them, that they can readily establish or re-establish contact, and that case managers will drop by from time to time to see how they are. At times, we will also tell clients that we can no longer work with them, that when they decide to do more for themselves, in accordance with their overt abilities to do so, we will re-engage with them.

We introduce these ideas here in order to share our own struggles with you, for in every instance mentioned above, we feel our own vulnerability and experience the uncertainty which accompanies an open-ended practice design. To illustrate this concept more clearly, in trying to embody the practice principles we have articulated, we turn over to the case managers and their supervisors the creative tasks of transforming principles into behaviors and evaluating the effectiveness of the practice. When we reach an impasse with a client, such as any of those described above, workers often experience the impasse as a sign of their own failure, a reaction which is the flip side of conventional 'victim blaming' which takes place when a client 'fails' to respond properly to one or another of the technologies employed by other mental health agencies. In this case, we try to use the same practice principles on ourselves that we employ with clients; elaboration of what has happened, connection of the feelings of the case managers to the events that have transpired, and examination of the interaction between the two dimensions of the situation. The effort is to share the frustration of impasse, to generate shared critical commentary, and to share the creative activity of producing a new practice. One method of helping to produce critical commentary as well as shared creative activity is the utilization of case management teams as an alternative to more isolated individual practice. Critical assessment of practice, support through periods of frustration, sharing of creative efforts to figure out new approaches to clients and peer supervision (in addition to regular, structured supervision) have been the outcome.

Case management is an enormously difficult and complex job. We have tried to show how its typical formulation is ridden with obstructions and contradiction, and how an alternative approach might be designed and implemented. We have argued that assuming the residual position of coordinator of services reduces the purpose and value of case management by reproducing the ex-patient as a passive, objectified consumer of services. In contrast, we have conveyed the focus of our advocacy/empowerment commitments to work with people toward becoming more active participants/producers of their social world. The move from passive consumer to more active producer signifies not only a shift in behavior in the social world, but a definite alteration in self-perception and self-judgment, a growing self-confidence restored to a person. Self-confidence gained through confrontation with an oppressive social reality and engagements in actions to transform this reality replace the self-contempt as characteristic of mental patient identity in a static world. We must continue the struggle to produce this type of development with people. In the process, our own development is assured. The dynamic of movement/development only occurs when the process is characterized by the dialogue and derived action that we have described and not short-circuited and stultified by 'professional' social role-defined communication and concern.

We move now to discuss the ways in which our practice approach can be developed in day programs of one type or another. From there, we will move on to a clearer description of the practice areas further removed from direct client contact, but equally centered in the same problem definition and practice theory.

CHAPTER 5

Day Programs

As the problem of emptying the hospitals became transformed into the problem of maintaining people in the community, the need for community-based program activities became apparent. Day programs of one type or another had been a formal part of community mental health policy since day hospital programming was required as one of the five stipulated services of the federally-funded community mental health centers program. Since then the number and variety of types of day programs have grown dramatically to include such program categories as day hospitals, training programs highlighting 'normalization' and/or 'socialization' skills, vocationally-oriented programs and psycho-social clubs.

It is not our intent to examine each type of program separately. Our focus will be on community-based programs for former patients with the understanding that funding agency guidelines and categories often limit or confine program development to restrictive activities – or, more likely, they appear to do this. We conjecture that the practice principles described in Chapter 2 can be introduced into at least some significant part of every type of community-based day program, whatever its formal program category. We know that we have used our conceptual framework and approach to practice in such program classifications as 'Coping Skills,' 'Competency Training,' 'Psycho-social Club' and even 'Case Management.' So while we do recognize the apparent boundaries set up by funding mechanisms, we also fully realize the actual flexibility available within each type of category.

Most former patients probably have been involved in a group-focused 'therapy' program of some kind, presumably while still inpatients. In these programs, as in community-based programs operated by most mental health service providers, the likelihood is that the conceptual model for implementing the activities involved was a medical-psychiatric approach. In program terms, this has meant that groups, both large and small, were premised on the assumption that the participants' behavior patterns, which reflect the social role of the mental patient, and their human identities were the same. In such groups people either learned to behave 'appropriately' or participated in condescending rituals directed at improving their 'functioning,' with this latter concept used to connote 'proper' behavior within the confines of the mental patient role.

Groups, especially from programs which focused on 'normalization' or 'socialization,' explicitly directed their attention to improved 'social functioning,' again constrained by what the program defined as appropriate to a mental patient operating at a quantitatively higher behavioral level. The patients then consumed available services and reproduced themselves as patients.

We arrive at an ironic situation: participating in such programs is almost always preferable to sitting in a ward or in an adult home, but the choice is based on the absence of something better. It also reaffirms the participants' infirmities by reproducing their diagnoses and the social system which assigns them. Pre-vocational programs do much the same, further and more overtly developing the 'as if' world of mental health agencies: the 'as if' aspect reflects the fact that programs often operate as if the substantive content of their program were real, 'as if' it were possible for a 45 year old man or woman with twenty-five years inpatient experience and the physical demeanor and income that comes with it could, after attending a pre-vocational program, progress through an occupational therapy program to a vocational therapy program to a vocational rehabilitation program to an on-the-job-training program, then enter the competitive labor market and live happily ever after. For their participation in these programs, patients and former patients are rewarded by staff and landlords, often with such tokens as certificates or such rewards as 'real' coffee, or being allowed to keep the trinkets which get produced from time to time. Our view is that these programs are typically infantilizing, disconnected from the concrete reality of either life on the ward or in the community and are therefore humiliating.

The results of participating in programs such as these, together with the dependency-producing behaviours of routine in the hospital, combine to produce the patterned interactions of mental patienthood. These behaviors clearly express the powerlessness and social status of invalidated people.

Quite obviously, in order to create a day program which embodies the concepts of advocacy/empowerment, we must present both a totally different program purpose and a set of activities which challenge the dependent/dominated social role of mental patients. Many of the same principles and ideas which we describe here will be applicable in the case management and other practice chapters, but there are some significant differences. For example, the vastly different circumstances of a program run within your own facility provide opportunities not available to clients who must rely on individual contact services delivered in the places where they live.

Having some control over the space where a program is run allows you to communicate something directly by the visual appearance of the program place. We have noticed that a number of programs seem to be decorated in ways communicating both infantilization of clients (juvenile pictures and smile faces) and/or rigid, dictatorial procedures such as huge, block-lettered schedules for daily activities and directives about such 'normalization' prerequisites as face washing and tooth brushing. Some other programs 'dress down,' usually because of lack of funds, and provide a more realistic atmosphere.

We believe that a significant amount of information should be made available which communicates not only who we are – brochures, announcements, etc. – but also what our perception is of the reasons why people are coming to a day program. For this reason, resource material is readily available and in public view: pamphlets covering legal rights and entitlements are everywhere, with emphasis on the former patient's status as a tenant most pronounced. Other information about entitlement benefits related to health care, Medicaid, vocational rehabilitation, etc., are available. Signs posted inform participants of any particular issues, meetings and/or visitors scheduled relating to legal rights and/or entitlements. Other posted information announces community events and/or organizations which might be of interest, reinforcing our belief that the former patient is indeed a citizen of his/her community. Active voter registration supports this view and reflects itself by postings of campaign meetings, notices of political activities of such organizations as anti-nuclear groups or women's groups, and procedural information about how to vote and get transportation to the polls. All of this material is reinforced in community meetings and the daily meetings of the various smaller groups which form the nucleus of the day program.

Since the program must be operated by the people who work there and those who participate in the program, the responsibilities for maintaining the program space are shared by both. We have no custodial staff, and so development of a work schedule to clean the rooms which are used for program activities is necessary. This schedule, too, is publicly posted and chores are assigned or voluntarily chosen, but in either case, what is to be done is designated as 'housework,' not given some mystified meaning such as learning a set of 'socialization skills.' Participation in the maintenance work of the place is done neither as a form of functional improvement and competition, nor on a reward system; rather, such work is expected of everyone with tasks assigned in some proximity to our estimate of each person's capacity. Where skills are involved, they are taught to new participants by those who are already familiar with what has to be done. Staff also does the same work, often together in work groups with participants, demonstrating that there is no absolute split between mental and physical labor. We want to make note of the fact that in this area, as in a number of others, similar behavioral acts – such as cleaning up, sweeping, etc. – carry with them different social meaning when the social relations of the people involved differ. We certainly are not trying either to romanticize custodial labor nor to mystify it. Rather, we want to be clear that labor that is done as shared necessary tasks without status or bosses, without deceit ('normalization skills') and domination, means something different than the same tasks performed under infantilizing or servile conditions. Things may look the same to outsiders, but be experienced very differently by participants.

Other visual aspects of our program include a bulletin board used by clients to post notices directly expressing their interests; a corner where the client-produced newsletter is posted and available to be taken home; and a posting of the different rooms is identified for service functions throughout the building. Since our program has a case management component, information about case management and the case managers' phone numbers also are posted prominently.

Another visual presentation of the program's basis can be developed jointly with the participants. It consists of taking photographs of various activities common to the program – cooking and/or eating, community meetings, small group meetings, outings etc. – and making

up posters which combine the photographs and descriptive statements about each activity with comments about it from the participants
who are shown in the photos. These posters are a record of what has
been done or is being done and can be an introduction to the program
for new members. The posters can be created and put up, as with much
of the other material described above, even in those circumstances
where use of program space is temporary and everything must be
removed after each program day. While visual displays may be
troublesome under these circumstances, the value of representing the
context and aspects of the shared experience is, we believe, well worth
the time involved.

Through the visual displays such as we have described, we hope to
communicate several themes to participants: that there are a set of
concrete problems permeating their social reality; that we recognize
the existence and complexity of these problems; that the problems are
social in nature (that is, that they are structural); and that the problems
are externally imposed and experienced in common. Housing, income, health and mental health care, and all other service sectors that
intersect and impact on clients' lives are identified visually to emphasize these themes. Reading materials related to legal rights, entitlements and grievance procedures (in written form, in a language
understandable by most elementary level readers) are readily available. In addition, clients experienced in dealing with various agencies
who are interested in working with other participants in relation to a
problem with a particular agency have their names posted. Clients are
also told that case managers are easily available and how to contact
them.

In addition to the material already mentioned, our program does a
great deal to develop community ties (more of which will be discussed
in Chapter 8). Obviously, being located in a neighborhood or a
community does not mean being from that area or of that group.
Mental health programs, or any program working with stigmatized
people, will often be regarded with fear and/or treated as an outsider in
any community or neighborhood in which it is located. In the case of
former patients, given the chaotic frenzy of the early years of deinstitutionalization and the frequent practice of dumping large numbers of
institutionalized ex-patients in communities ill prepared to handle
them and unprepared to provide services for them, community antagonism is not unusual. Couple to this more recent demand for non-
profit community half-way houses and free use of eminent domain by

state government to relocate other patients and we see exacerbated fears about community property values. Any day program endeavor that does not try to build positive community ties is in jeopardy at any time tensions arise. Therefore, we make efforts to communicate with community groups, churches, civic organizations, etc. We invite them to come to our program, either to talk about their church or organization, to drop in to say hello, or to approach us with some potential volunteer effort. When notices of community sponsored activity are identified, a representative of the sponsoring group is asked to come and personally invite the participants to attend.

Programming for us consists of a variety of activities, some constant, some transitory or short term, and some which are unanticipated or spontaneous. One activity which will occur at the beginning of every program day and, if necessary, again that same day if staff feel some critical issue has come up, is the community meeting. Every day there will be groups meeting, some ongoing, others more short term, some ad hoc. Some groups have an open membership, some have a specific target membership and are closed to everyone else. For those few individuals who seem unable to meet in groups, or to interact socially, no pressure is put on except for required attendance at the community meeting, some contribution to the maintenance work, and some participation in food preparation and/or clean-up, if the person partakes of what is offered.

Community meetings, another common activity of most day programs, have three purposes in our program: daily activities are reviewed including identifying the groups (by time and place) occurring that day; a summary, thematizing the focus of each group and its current substantive area will be presented and brief comments elicited; and any information that people have learned regarding resources, benefits or services will be shared. In addition, people representing different agencies or programs are often invited to the community meeting to describe their agency's function, how it can be used, and to answer questions that the participants may have about it. Clients who have experience with any service or agency are asked to share their experiences with others. Again, the issues discussed at the community meetings are grounded in daily life.

The review of the thematic content of specific groups is done to keep everyone informed about what is happening and to elicit perspectives from people outside the specific groups about what they are hearing. In addition, this review validates the group members by sharing their experiences and perceptions thematically with the group at large. We are trying to present both the substantive issues of daily life and the process of struggle (as expressed through group participation) as critical aspects of personal development. To do this we represent positive activities and painful experiences back to everyone in order to help people see and feel the reconnection of their experience to the harsh conditions which govern daily life, and to the pain of the past intrusions into that life by hospitalization. We also encourage people to share positive feelings and experiences of self-confidence that arise in the course of ongoing struggles.

Social development, which we also refer to as shared empowerment, emerges as people, at whatever level or pace each person is able to engage, come to some understanding that their personal lives are also expressions of social reality, of shared economic deprivation, of shared powerlessness. Equally important, as a complementary dimension to our process of 'recontextualization' or reconnection, is the process of talking openly at the community meeting about how one has experienced participation in programs, advocacy activities, etc. This process usually involves a person describing what he/she was trying to do (e.g., get the homeowner to turn the Medicaid card over to her/him) and what was felt during each step of the process. People's feelings and objectively identifiable conditions are thus increasingly presented as interwoven, a practice that carries over into all other groups. Participants are invited to share their similar experiences or similar feelings in relation to the conditions being described ('Has anyone been through a situation like X has just described?' 'Are X's feelings familiar to any of you?'). Our purpose is to create a context where emerging critical ideas are joined to positive emotional experience and the process of struggle.

We believe that the common base of people's experience is undermined in daily life, in the everyday ideology of social life and, in heightened form, for anyone with experience in the mental health system because of its saturation by an individual defect form of problem definition. Therefore, we try to develop group activities whenever we can. Groups are formed either out of direct concerns that participants bring to us, issues which case managers bring to us and to the participants (through presentations at community meetings), or through staff-initiated stimuli.

An example of a group developed directly in response to participants' concerns would be an ad hoc group of residents from an SRO who wanted to meet to discuss recurring problems at their place of residence. These problems were presented initially as a series of complaints or gripes at a community meeting. The people were organized into an ad hoc group by a staff member who suggested that anyone concerned with the issues being discussed might want to explore them in greater depth. Residents of the SRO were joined by a few other participants who lived in different SRO housing to explore the facts, to focus attention on their status as tenants, and to formulate some concept of what could be done. This group eventually decided to invite community people in to hear the issues and to join in some cooperative strategy. Case managers familiar with the people and the SROs can also be invited to participate as group members or as resource persons.

Case manager initiated groups also have formed in response to issues usually associated with a service system. For example, the SSI decertification scandal, the HEAP (Home Energy Assistance Program) and certain state-supported tax rebate allowances available to clients have all produced ad hoc groups which included case managers and day program staff. These groups were often very large because they dealt with issues related to income or resources that were tangible rather than service-centered.

Staff-initiated groups tend to be those which deal with more long term problems or very short term situations. Examples of longer term groups which staff have started, after representations of people's comments and concerns, include a health group, a women's group and a group for adult home residents focused on rights and entitlements related to the legal status of their type of residence. Short term groups have been convened to discuss plans for a holiday party, to develop a method for distributing donations of clothes and to examine some problems which developed between the people responsible for meal preparation on a given evening. As with the other types of groups, each of these was begun with a presentation at a community meeting and an open discussion of issues in that forum. In every case, the formation of a group was presented as one possible response to the issues made public at the community meeting.

The groups which we believe are conducive to social development are those which contemplate and reflect on aspects of daily life. Our purpose is to allow people to examine critically the conditions of life, the feelings they have about themselves and their situation, and the potential actions that can emerge. Any number of groups can exist and we mention several here which we have found effective. A health group, meeting to discuss people's experiences with current and past health care, can discuss how people can best present themselves to physicians, and what to expect from their doctors, what their legal rights are (e.g., getting a second opinion or choosing the doctor they want to see, in spite of the existence of the landlord's 'house' doctor), and what their feelings are about dealing with health care personnel. A women's group might discuss women's past and present experiences with sexual abuse and/or harassment, treatment by hospital and residence staff or other issues which reflect sexist domination. A drug information group might explore issues related to informed consent, the right to know about medication and/or to refuse it, and the right to know about side effects of drugs. In addition, the group might go over strategies for relating to mental health clinic psychiatrists in ways that give the members more control over their own bodies. A younger people's group might discuss the particular experience of being relatively young (twenty to thirty-seven for present members) and 'stuck' in the role of ex-patient.

The more enduring groups have several related foci: to deal with or raise problems which occur routinely and generally are accepted as part of a reality which the participants initially perceive to be beyond their knowledge and out of their control; to attempt to reconnect systematically the realm of subjectivity (feelings and self-perception) to objective circumstances; to introduce material which asserts the participants' dignity as human beings and thus to pose a challenge to the mental patient role. In all of these endeavors, the attempt is made to build collectivity by identifying the common bases for ongoing struggle.

Groups of a shorter duration do not differ significantly in their purposes from those described above. While groups of shorter duration have the same process commitments, they may have a more precise focus such as voter registration, a legal case involving one or more participants or a group made up of the residents of a particular home or type of residence who have got together to discuss a problem related to their specific living circumstances. Whatever the particulars of the group, the practice principles, the struggle to redefine problems and the effort to move from tacit acquiescence (through critical reflection) to strategic contemplation of action remains the same. Similarly, the process of helping people to develop an elaboration of their perceptions and feelings about these perceptions, of thematizing the descriptive content for representation, of reflecting on emerging thematic patterns, and using these patterns to problematize and plan action schema occur in all groups.

We ask that either a group leader/staff member or a participant briefly summarize/thematize the activities and interactions of each group at least once a week at the community meeting. We also encourage each group to write a brief column in our newsletter as another way of sharing with other participants the activities and thematic content emerging from the group. We see the process of writing the narrative as a way of taking valid and valuable activity and experience from the realm of the subjective and introducing it into the larger, more objective context as a statement about people's capacities, insights and potential or actual resourcefulness to one another. Reinforcement of the interaction of subjectivity with objectivity, of the validity of human struggle, of the emerging nature of both group bonds and humanized problematization all form prevailing reasons for these practices. The verbal and written group summaries also regularly remind people that they are being taken seriously, that their struggles are serious ones well worth making public and receiving others' positive attention. The static life of the inpatient, replicated in the monotonous, repetitive existence of the after-care patient residing in profit-settings, is posed as a problem through this process of continuity of participation, serious deliberation of issues with social meaning and development of strategic interventions.

Other, less formal groups also occur. Groups have formed to do exercise, to expand cooking and knowledge of foods, to put the newsletter together, to produce a garden, etc. And, while these groups seem to be less 'heavy,' less overtly connected to our conceptual framework for defining problems, they still retain the same ideological orientation. The emphasis is on participation rather than performance, on doing things actively together rather than on competitive individual functioning. The effort extended by a reticent participant is supported as vigorously as any exceptionally well done function. Through the groups which require less verbal interaction we hope to involve people less certain of themselves, less confident in their ability to communicate, more frightened about alternatives to the mental patient role behaviors that they have been coerced into seeing as synonymous with themselves.

These less verbal groups are frequently characterized by a great deal of fun, as people share activity together without fear of assessment on either a patient-role functional scale or even a personal level of success or failure. The mixture of people who participate in such groups covers the range of members, from younger people with multiple short-term hospitalizations to older folks who spent one very long period incarcerated. With staff leadership acting to criticize competitive routines frequently introduced by younger, newer participants, the groups function well. The groups are encouraged to reflect critically on their shared activity, the failure-free context for doing it, and its comparative relation to the conditions of their daily lives. For example, an exercise group or a cooking group might talk about how they felt exercising or cooking together and then might discuss whether the same activity could occur in the profit-based homes where they live. Such a discussion allows group participants to reflect on the positive activity experienced in the group and then to use their reflection to look at other parts of their daily lives critically. These groups also report at the community meetings and in the newsletter. Participation in these groups is not accorded second class status, since the practice principles are not rooted in a therapeutic model which gives primacy to more verbal, sociable people.

In the case of every group, the basis for the existence of the group comes from the daily lives and experiences of the participants. Initiation of a group may come either from staff or participants, with staff providing leadership in the initial period of the groups. As program participants become accustomed to being taken seriously, as they start to see different ways of perceiving their situations, ideas for groups slowly emerge. The focus of any new group thus reflects some readily identifiable dimension of people's daily experience. The health group, for example, began as a result of a spontaneous discussion at a community meeting. One person mentioned that the physician selected by the homeowner was coming that week and she did not like him. Upon elaboration, it turned out that all of the owners of the local adult homes had similar arrangements with the same doctor, who received Medicaid reimbursement for his 'services.' Very few people liked him or felt they received good treatment. Issues related to choosing a physician, securing second medical opinions, controlling Medicaid cards, defining 'good' treatment, responding to doctors one does not like, etc., all emerged quickly as real issues. When the sequence of complaints was over, the idea of organizing a group to deal with health-related issues and experiences became self-evident. The idea for the group arose from one person feeling safe enough to complain publicly, and staff pursuing the substance and serious basis of the issue vigorously.

When information is communicated to us privately or problems are made known to us by case managers, we will ask either an individual or a case manager to come forward at a community meeting to share his/her perception or feelings. If the participant refuses, or will not release the case manager or other staff member to do it, staff will ask if they can introduce the issue, with or without the participant's name. If we are refused, staff will not raise the concern. What they will do, in instances such as this, is attempt to identify a larger theme into which the particular matter fits, and see if there might be a way to introduce public discussion of that theme as a way of including the issue and the person who brought it to us in a more public arena.

A participant has been complaining to the staff that the home-owner has not given her enough money for the previous two months. The issue and the client's perception of what is going on have been elaborated. The client is afraid to talk to other residents to learn if they, too, are being exploited. She is frightened about taking any action, including bringing up the issue at the day program because other residents who have complained in the past were rehospitalized. Since income from SSI is regulated by both SSI and the State Department of Social Services, discussion of either or both of these sets of agencies and their regulations will encompass the concerns without identifying her by name. Workers from either SSI, the state regulatory agency and/or a legal services program can be invited in to address the community meeting about the issue. Group activity, including or apart from the visitors, can be proposed and introduced at the very least, the concerns of the client can be elaborated in a public arena, support for her feelings can be elicited from 'legitimated' sources, and identification with her fears can be generated by asking people about how they would feel in a situation where they knew their money was being taken by some one as powerful as their landlord.

Turning privately felt issues into publicly visible forums is simultaneously threatening and validating: it threatens the person with exposure, either as being 'crazy' or as saying something antagonistic about a power holder (landlord, clinic, doctor, physician, etc.); and, on the other hand, it connects the person with others experiencing similar feelings, thus objectifying what was previously subjective, and legitimating the concern as concretely valid, while also allowing the person to experience her/himself in a leadership capacity. When we recall that our clients have been invalidated by the psychiatric system, and have lost all confidence in themselves as commentators on their own social experience, the process of supporting public exposure and bringing up personal perceptions of issues is vital. But, as we have indicated, such public statements can also be problematic: for example, another participant tells the owner or manager of the adult home about complaints being made by another resident. Even this type of problem situation, however, can be used positively: such a situation can be used to prompt a discussion at a community meeting about communicating strategically, about whose interests are served by 'leaking' critical comments about home owners, etc. Talking about an issue as threatening, as 'leaked' information, publicly makes the problem a common situation to be addressed strategically and shows how a common occurrence can be used to explore some of the political dimensions of daily life, both in relation to content and process. Public discussion converts privately felt, subjectively perceived feelings and thoughts into another arena – a potentially political analytic context which converts submerged beliefs into actionable deliberation.

Transforming ideas and feelings about daily life, about activities and people, or about one's participation in the program itself into shared concerns and possible social criticisms provides a form of validation for most participants which they have been denied during their contact with the mental health system. As a mental patient, rewards have been for behaviors and performed acts – measures of social function – that have served the interests of others. In our program, we are trying to do very much the opposite: we are trying to allow people to express and experience themselves as people engaged in some type of struggle to know more about their world in order to act on it. Crucial to this effort is the capacity to express what one believes to be true, and to be respected for the communication. Respect, obviously, does not mean non-critical acceptance of what is said, but rather stands for the right of the person to share her/his perceptions or feelings and to have these perceptions and feelings taken seriously.

The issue of involving people in decision making about their own activities within a program illustrates this theme of taking people more seriously. Freire talks about 'false charity' being an ingratiating stance taken towards the oppressed which refuses to deal with the causes of their oppression. Many vocational socialization programs manifest such 'false charity.' Even in psycho-social club programs the same tendency, in a somewhat hidden form, can be seen as well. In psycho-social clubs, the effort is made to involve patients, usually referred to as 'members' (to appear to avoid being associated with the underlying medical mode), in program planning by asking them what they want to do. The response, of course, reflects prevailing mental patient role identity learned during periods of hospitalization and medical model after-care. Ex-patients' responses are usually made up of those things which the people, as 'mental patients,' have enjoyed: picnics, shopping trips, arts and crafts, etc. These then become the activities of the club, if the staff wants to do them, and all are mystified into thinking that some democratic participation has occurred. What really has transpired is the reproduction of domination in a benevolent form. The identities of both patients and staff are reconfirmed through false charity and false participation since the solicitation about preferred activity is in fact a closed-ended question confined to those interactions which reproduce the invalid existence of the mental patient as the reciprocal function of the legitimate staff persons. Allowable activities, for example, are unlikely to include a topic such as discussion of the conflict of interest that exists when program staff are part of a 'team' that includes the homeowner or manager of an SRO.

When people tell you that they want to do childish things constantly (since there is no absolute negative in an occasional picnic) and the scope of their expressed concerns is play-like, it tells you what they think about themselves, about their low level of self-confidence as people and something about how they perceive you. They are 'playing it safe.' Most club programs provide a setting suggesting the appropriateness of such safe, child-like activities. Ours does not – the purpose of our program is not replication of existing power relations, exploitative arrangements and common forms of manipulation. Our program consciously works against sustaining oppression. Coming to a program committed to advocacy/empowerment does involve a risk: the power holders in our clients' lives – homeowners/managers, medical model clinics, etc. – often attempt to intimidate people and prevent their involvement in our program. Additionally, clients can perceive a risk to challenge one's 'safe identity' as a mental patient, even if such an identity has proven to be thoroughly confining. But, we feel we have no choice except to challenge the 'safety' of both the mental patient caretaker system and the identity which such a system reinforces.

Obviously, simply to challenge this system with competing rhetoric is absurd and self-defeating. Many mental health agencies are challenged by our differing concepts of relationships with people, by our concept of confidentiality, by commitments to participants which are expressed in our refusal to participate in the agency-based treatment teams or in the agency-homeowner alliances and by our concept of programming. To illustrate this point at some length, we return to the common request to go on a shopping trip.

Where a positive response to such a request might involve taking a group of ex-patients on a hospital bus or clinic van to some shopping center, our approach does not. We begin with a planning session that has a series of tasks: first, the plotting of a course on public transportation. Bus schedules and maps are scrutinized, with people trying to locate where they live and figure out the closest bus stop (few, if any people placed in our geographic area by the state hospitals have any familiarity with the community). From a group discussion of maps and bus schedules, we can learn other important information, for example, who can read and who may have eye problems (many people have had eye damage caused by medication and/or neglect).

Identifying eye damage may produce a discussion of eye care received while in the hospital or at present: such discussions have resulted in more than one person getting glasses. Since Medicaid cards are necessary to obtain both eye care and reduced bus tokens, we may proceed with a discussion about 'house doctors' – the quality of care delivered and who benefits from such an arrangement. People may also be encouraged to continue this health-related discussion with the case managers and may also be reminded that the ongoing health group is a place where such issues can be explored in more depth. As the planning moves ahead, the issue of money to spend on the trip may be used to trigger a discussion of SSI cheques, personal allowance regulations and how money is handled in the homes where people live. People may want to talk about having more control over their money and the possibility of opening a personal bank account may be discussed. Thus, a simple shopping trip may very easily serve as a catalyst for discussion of some of the most important issues and themes in people's lives. A typical 'mental patient event' has been transformed into an ongoing, problem-identifying process directed towards critical reflection on daily life and potential action to change it.

Commitments to a similar process can be found in food preparation and eating together. Again, rather than produce snacks and meals as some type of 'socialization' skill or performance of normalized routine that forces people to be assessed or to compete with each other over best behaviors or best jobs, snacks and meals are prepared and eaten as a process of shared participation and work. Preparing food and setting up for a meal are seen as common activities containing an opportunity for many people to contribute to the community of participants and staff sharing the food. Tasks are broken down so as to allow everyone to take part (not necessarily on every day, but regularly), and equal value is attached to each activity to maximize participation and minimize competition and condescension. People are given some control over the process of production and no division occurs between staff and participants that reflects a permanent division between mental and physical labor. Participants are asked to choose the tasks they want to do, with staff overseeing the distribution and assuring that everyone takes part. For people who refuse, discussion with staff ensues to determine why they are not involved. People's belief that they do not have any useful ability as 'mental patients' is challenged constantly and gradually most people are able to contribute in some way. Others who continue to refuse to produce socially useful and necessary labor – sharing in task production around meals – are told that they cannot benefit from the labor of others and are not permitted to share in the food. If the same behavior carries over to cleaning up the rooms used in the program, the person is asked not to return until she/he is ready to produce her/his share of the labor necessary to operate the program.

We have learned that simple nutritious meals can be prepared easily; that cooking and/or taking part in setting or cleaning up offers multiple opportunities for engaging people in socially useful activity; that efforts to engage people in shared tasks offer excellent opportunities for talking with people about past experiences with work; and that people who are often reluctant to talk in community meetings and/or smaller groups can often be engaged through shared task production. We see similar positive outcomes in the sharing of the meal. There is a marked difference between people who have attended the program for some time and newcomers at mealtime. We have small tables, seating six to ten people, where food is served 'family style' whenever possible. Almost inevitably newcomers will take the serving plate first and dish out far more than their share, leaving everyone else whatever is left. Participants are quite familiar with this behavior and readily engage the offender in a critical discussion, albeit at times rather heated. The point about individual accumulation versus shared benefits is made quite directly and continuously. The result of this process, where food is shared in much the same manner as the tasks necessary to produce it, is a far more humanized environment than their past or present living situation. The benefits gained by including meal preparation in a day program outweigh the problems of logistics as long as this activity, like others, is viewed as a process of helping people to identify and understand better the dominant themes in their lives. The entire process can also involve trips to buy the food, to plan and prepare for shopping, to budget and to learn to develop collective schemes. It can be as simple as making soup or as complex as trying to get homeowners to pay for it.

Food preparation for a full meal need not be done every day for cost containment reasons as well as not having to bring a facility up to health and safety code requirements for a restaurant. Preparing simple nutritious foods, such as soups and healthy breads, can be a meaningful social activity as well as a food supplement. Producing an evening meal once a week also brings people out at night and attracts some people who attend other day programs.

The issue of paying for food can also be introduced as a problem, even when programs have food costs included in their budgets. Many people living on SSI pay their landlords for both food and rent. Therefore, they can legally ask for box lunches or the equivalent in cash for any meals that they miss in the home. These people may authorize the project staff to ask for a payment in direct proportion to the number of people from each facility who attend the program when meals are served. Even if no collection from homeowners is actually done, participants can benefit from a community meeting where this issue is elaborated: they hear about their SSI cheques; they learn about how funds for room and board are calculated; they learn that their landlords are business people who make a profit from their housing; and the participants learn another way of understanding themselves – as rent-paying tenants rather than mental patients being 'treated.'

Advocacy/empowerment practice – concepts of leadership

We turn now from a discussion of the nature of programs to a discussion of our concept of leadership and of staff participation and responsibilities. Properly trained and supported staff are central to any program. When a program turns away from dominant ideology and seeks to develop an advocacy/empowerment approach to practice, the significance of prior training of staff drops at the same time as the priority of in-service training and support systems rises. The reason for devaluing formal training is simply that we know of no formal academic degree program in which our theoretical position is communicated in either its content or learning theory. While we do not discount people with academic credentials, neither do we overestimate their potential value. In-service training, therefore, takes on a value and import beyond what is generally thought to be necessary to run most programs. This concept, too, has its basis in ideological difference: most agencies expect people to fill job slots where tasks and functions are rather rigidly defined. We seek people who have some commitment to producing, rather than simply reproducing, the activities in which they are engaged. Consequently, our in-service training time is devoted to exploration of theory and practice principles, to critical reflection of how these matters are applied in practice, and to creating a problem-posing practice. We hope to develop staff solidarity through building trust, sharing as much of the decision making and policy setting among all staff as we can, and through critical examinations of issues which arise in the course of practice. We hope to communicate to staff that our concept of practice is based on the set of critical principles discussed above, and not on a set of specific behaviors. This complicated point means that while practice principles and some particular activities (e.g. community meetings) are appreciated and expected, figuring out exactly how to operationalize these principles rests largely with line staff and supervisors. Therefore, in-service training tends to focus or refocus on principles and problem situations defined by staff as needing attention.

As we turn now to more particular responsibilities, we ask that the reader turn back to the practice theory chapter and review the issues and principles which we have extrapolated from Freire's work. We believe that a review of the theoretical thrust of our work will best inform the more particularized material which appears below.

Leadership requires a developing understanding of how our program defines the problems confronted by the former patient population (see Chapter 1). Leadership also requires the ability to allow the client group to teach workers about their reality in terms of perception and experience, and for staff to be prepared to enter this realm of perception and feeling as best they can. So, additionally, staff have to be willing to be uncertain, to find struggling to identify problems and interim strategies more self-sustaining than reproducing professional

roles and locating personal validity through domination or conventional legitimation.

Understanding our theoretical framework for problem definition is
essential to being able to communicate with former patients in some
manner other than condescension. A primary leadership responsibility
here, as in case management, is to produce elaborations of people's
thoughts and feelings about whatever content is presented. Elaboration, rather than simply pushing the person to go on talking without
purpose, allows us to learn more about the person's perception of
reality and his/her feelings about it. Elaboration communicates several
things: that we are taking the person absolutely seriously; that she/he
has something of value to say about the social world and her/his view of
their place in it: that the feelings she/he has are real and very much
different from the ruminations of a 'crazy' person. Primary emphasis is
put on stimulating elaborated but focused discussions, and looking at
what has been said in relation to contributions made by other participants. This process is an attempt to assist people to see and feel their
common bases or foundations for collectivity. Staff are required to be
able to use the theory to thematize, that is to understand the specific
content or behavior of what is presented at a descriptive level, bringing
these descriptive accounts into sharper focus. It is the first level of
abstraction – the theme – which is eventually referred back or represented to people for their critical reflection. The themes come from
our theoretical/critical analysis of the causes of reality and reflect our
commitments to social change.

The themes developed after extensive descriptive elaboration are
meant to illuminate the concealed meaning in much of what is being
said and/or how it is being said. The thematic content of the descriptive
material is deciphered through understanding that the hidden basis of
such material is to be found in the existence of oppression/
powerlessness, domination/submissiveness, exploitation/helplessness,
or manipulation/self-contempt. The ideology of the society, exacerbated by the particular form of the psychiatric model and its associated
behaviors for staff and mental patients, excludes any of these themes
from conceptual or emotional legitimacy or validation. In the presentation of the compelling themes ('generative themes' in Freire's
terms) above, we have identified the conceptual dimension as well as
the emotional dimension for each theme. We believe that the people
who talk to us do so either through these themes or about them or
both. But, because the substantive content and the emotional experi-

ence have no conceptual validity, the true content is disguised by and distorted by mainstream ideology and 'safe' mental patient behavior. It is our task to work through both to create clarity about the thematic patterns that are grounded in objective conditions reflecting oppression, domination, exploitation and manipulation, and their derived emotional content of powerlessness, helplessness, self-contempt and submission.

Obviously, these themes cannot be introduced immediately. What is required is to develop a strategy that builds upon interim derivative concepts much closer to daily life. Such concepts flow from the reality of the ex-patients' lives and have been discussed above. The housing situation for most ex-patients allows for transformation from a treatment context into a landlord-tenant context (see Chapter 6); voter registration allows for transformation from mental patient into citizen; legal rights and entitlements promote possibilities for other transformations from mental patient into social being; health care needs, differentiated from mental health, offer opportunities for similar changes in self-perception, etc. All of these arenas logically flow from our dedication to the concrete social life of the person as the basis for recontextualizing their experience, for reestablishing the relation between concrete-historical-material conditions and subjectivity.

Injected into this framework, as an elaboration of it, is the projected impact of mental patient status on identity, on undermining of self-confidence. The concept of the person oppressed by the interaction of the objective conditions of the present, with the subjective domination from past and present mental patient role coercion, connects the compelling themes discussed above to the experience of daily life. The interim thematic content discussed above thus reflects the substantive concerns and behaviors of ex-patients expressed through our concept of the causes of reality and its impact on people. The interim thematic content reflects Freire's concepts of limit-situations and problem-posing as primary strategic activities.

The following is an example from our experience of the use of interim thematic content to develop critical consciousness. A group of people who ordinarily do not take an active role in community meetings or smaller groups has become involved in an exercise group initiated by one of the staff. The exercises are not overtly strenuous as several of the members are older people who have some difficulty with coordination. Members are asked to design exercise movements which all can do, including two people who must remain seated. Amid the laughter, people cooperate with each other in trying to do whatever any member suggests. After several meetings, people describe how good it feels to do something physical and fun. This is used immediately by the staff person to develop some elaboration about past and present experiences doing activities that were active and fun. Soon thereafter, in representing what the people had said about the experience in the group, the leader asks people to compare their experience in the group with daily living in the homes. People talk about the monotony of the routine of daily life as sedentary, passive, with people watching TV or sitting smoking. There follows a discussion of why this occurs, about whose interests were served by such docility, about why the landlord/managers prefer passive, domesticated residents. The results of these discussions, coupled with demonstrations of newly created exercises, were presented at a community meeting and written up in the newsletter. The discussion issues transcended the particular group and generated extensive response in the larger group. The people who actively created the issue, brought to a greater level of understanding by the leader's skill in interim thematization, felt strengthened through the experience and joined with one or two others to discuss possibilities for creating some exercise groups in the places where they live. Some of the people are now more likely to join other groups which have talking as their primary medium of communication, thus broadening their forums of participation, while bringing to the more verbally active people another arena in which the themes that they have been deliberating can be connected to the new material as a thematic pattern, the basis for problematization.

The voter registration group offers another example of staff leadership and thematization. The group had previously filled out voter registration forms, received their formal cards, and discussed what these activities meant to them. The group then began ongoing discussion about a coming election. When a participant mentioned asking local candidates to come to the program, this idea was agreed upon by the group and referred to the community meeting. At this meeting, voter registration cards were shown and people were asked how they felt about having their own cards. After a discussion, a collective letter of invitation was sent to a candidate for the state legislature who knew our program quite well and who we believed would come to talk to this particular group of voters. Participants who were not part of the voter group were invited to join in preparation for the coming visit. This produced the equivalent of a civics class for several weeks as members had to sort out what kinds of issues and questions were most appropriate to ask a candidate for state legislative office. The meeting went very well as questions both appropriate to the visit and some beyond the visitor's comprehension were brought up. After the visitor left, the staff person represented the issues which seemed to be of greatest concern in an interim thematic form: people wanted to know more about the state role in SSI, in recertification hearings, and in monitoring the regulatory agency charged with inspecting and evaluating adult homes. The operative theme was the desire people had to know more about the legal parameters governing their living situations and how these guidelines related to the particular places where each of them lived. After careful and extensive review of the issues expressed and represented as interim themes, the voter group decided to transform its purpose, after the election, to following up on the thematic issues. This turn of events reflects how thematic involvement and representation can lead to thematic patterns and to problematizing – to setting forth a new formulation of a problem or series of problems amenable to action by the participants.

In the examples of both groups, the leaders continually moved from the content of the group's activities or its discussions to eliciting how people felt about the related issues; or, conversely, the leaders helped participants move from expressions of feelings to the situations governing people's lives. In both groups, for instance, people became very angry from time to time at issues such as the sedentary nature of life in the homes or about the numerous violations of regulations existing in the adult homes. These feelings were acknowledged, people were encouraged to tell others how they felt, and the objective bases for the feelings were identified. Reconnecting this anger to the powerless position people were in vis-à-vis landlords and managers transformed a subjective experience, felt in isolation from others, into a shared experience of validation which others could acknowledge and support. It also created the possibility for objective reflection on the situations described and the possibilities of action (see Chapter 6).

During the process of each group, every contribution was acknowledged by the leader who mentioned the name of the contributor. In addition, individual statements were probed for elaboration and the contributions of each person were summarized by the leader at the end of each session. This summary was written up by the leader and represented to the group members at the next session. A member was then elected to report back to the community meeting and other members self-selected to join the leader to write a brief column covering group activities for the newsletter. People's contributions are publicly acknowledged, repeated aloud, stated at public meetings and converted into themes which appear in print. These activities provide for an uncustomary continuity, for being taken seriously and for sharing struggle in broader circles.

Other people who are unable or unwilling to join groups, or who come to them but cannot or will not focus on the group's area of concern, are invited to join in ongoing activity, but are not permitted to obstruct it. When interruptions occur in meetings, those causing the problem are confronted immediately by staff, if not by other participants, and stopped, even if such action requires asking someone to leave. This part of the process is also critically examined by staff and participants and not omitted from summaries. People in some form of crisis are attended to, but not allowed to demand total concentration from everyone.

Staff members must understand our theoretical perspective in order to take responsibility for initiating groups as vehicles for critical learning and reflection. Opportunities for participation and for eventual action are created by group leaders who can actively employ thematization. Developing patterns among the themes presented and representing the thematic patterns to participants also clearly requires thorough understanding of the theory involved in both problem definition and practice. Introducing themes or thematic patterns requires a sense of the validity of problem-posing rather than problem-solving as a form of practice. The tasks ultimately lead to this level – can we figure out a way of producing critical dialogue that will lead to some aspect of daily life being understood strategically? Can we stimulate and sustain a dialogue with people that will allow them to problematize some aspect of their static, controlled lives, and in the process come to see themselves as valid human beings? And, for staff, can they trust themselves and the people they work with enough to allow this process to develop, to support the process and the people even though the outcome is not predetermined and contained by staff needs?

There is a problem of ongoing concern to both day program workers and case managers: how to deal with issues which cannot be solved by working with clients directly, or which require some immediate responses before a strategy for action can be worked out with the client. Committed as we are to issues coming from the lives of the people, we want to involve the people in actions which will affect their lives. This is not a problem in case advocacy situations: action goes only as far and as fast as the client authorizes, with the full meaning of informed consent serving as the context. But, there are other times when we will act without full client involvement, particularly when we are dealing with issues beyond case advocacy. Two examples of measures which came from clients' lives and were converted into legislative action will be discussed in Chapter 6. Other types of issues get acted upon with varying degrees of client involvement: interagency meetings and meetings with community organizations are used to advocate for positions on various issues. The degree of client participation is worked out by staff and the results of such meetings are reflected back to clients at community meetings. Some examples of issues and levels of client participation include the following:

1 Some of our clients who are residents of a local SRO hotel complain bitterly about management. Their attempts to organize fall apart regularly because over 50 per cent of the SRO residents are alcoholic, dependent upon the owner and extremely unreliable when it comes to organizing. We consult with our participants about involving the local civic association, a close ally of our program. They approve and we move foward to mobilize support from the civic association. The civic association informs the owner that they will make sure that building code enforcement is done properly and unless the landlord brings the building into compliance, the civic association will organize townspeople to throw him out.

2 We offer our support as friends of the court to a legal program litigating a suit involving adult home residents against the State Department of Social Services.

3 We file formal complaint reports with the adult home regulatory agency whenever we are aware of violations. We inform clients of this action as it occurs. We push for litigation on any issue whenever possible, but this is difficult because a client must be the actual formal complainant.

4 We continually put forth our definition of confidentiality in interagency battles with the state hospital and psychiatric after-care clinic. We inform clients of these interactions, but indicate that we will not compromise our position on this issue regardless of what the policy decision on the matter is by the mental health system.

In addition, we try to keep clients regularly informed on any issue which has come up and become part of another political arena, as we will show with regard to our legislative examples in Chapter 6. We do want to note, however, that we must remember to keep the clients at the center of any action which can directly affect them and in which there might be any risk to them. In these matters, the decisions to be made are at all times fully theirs.

We close this chapter by raising two concerns which we believe require program attention: the policy of inclusion/exclusion of people from groups within the program, and how to respond to people who leave the program without any notice. The first question is more problematic: excluding people from groups (perhaps other than a women's group) communicates judgments about those excluded which are the exact contradiction of what we want people to feel in our program. On the other hand, leaving all small group membership open almost always means that individual group development is slowed or stultified by occasional participants who really have no particular interest in the group, but attend for the day because they have nothing better to entertain them. This type of situation always brings about disruption, because the person has to be filled in on what had been going on, or because she/he does not understand what the group is doing, or because she/he feels like talking that day, but not about any topic related to the group's purpose. Staff efforts to control interlopers or 'day trippers,' even where fully successful, disrupt the process of the group. Our view, tentatively formed, is to try to put together groups whose members are either initially self-selected or organized by staff in response to particular expressed interests or problems. These might include women's activities, younger people's struggles, a health group with people already quite familiar with major issues, another health group for people more submerged in daily life. Whether a group is self-selected or staff-initiated, the process must be made clear to everyone at a community meeting, so that discussion is possible and membership in any particular group is not mystified and accorded some special status.

For people who drop out of the program, we believe it necessary to conduct a carefully designed follow-up interview. Staff must be polled to learn what information they might have about why the person left. Furthermore, a staff member with a good relationship to the client is assigned the task of doing the follow-up interview. The purpose of this interview is to gain clarity about why the client has chosen to leave the program and to let the person know that we are not judging the decision, but only wanting to learn from it. Were there criticisms of the program? Were needs being met? Were there unfair practices going on? Criticism of the program can be expressed verbally or behaviorally. We want to allow the person dropping out the possibility for delivering criticism in a more targeted manner than their simple departure can communicate.

Summarizing, the common principles of practice we have tried to communicate are:

1 The prerequisite of understanding how to redefine clients' problems as a conscious component of practice. This social-being orientation allows us to see clients not just as mental patients incapable of any action on their own, but as oppressed people who endure both objectively grounded domination, poverty and powerlessness and subjective invalidation as well. These constitute what we have called the 'compelling themes' of daily life.

2 The struggle to generate dialogue with each person, thus posing a challenge to the person's mental patient identity. This process is done by listening critically to the complaints and problems presented, by introducing into the communication a real interest in having the person elaborate perceptions and feelings, and by seeking to reconnect or 'recontextualize' feelings/perceptions to objective and understandable circumstances.

3 After supporting sequential elaboration, and seeking to connect people to one another, seeking to help people move beyond the descriptions of reality to an understanding of its causes.

4 The struggle to gain causal understanding of clients' descriptive material by creating interim themes out of the descriptive material based on our critical understanding of the reality shared by our clients. We use this critical understanding to represent material back to the people that they have shared with us, filtered through our critical perspective as embodied in the interim themes we choose.

5 After elaborating the themes, we again seek the opportunity to synthesize discussion, identify thematic patterns and attempt to reformulate problems. This process is referred to as problematization, the arriving at new problem definitions through thematic dialogue.

6 Having come to new understandings of problem situations, new

action strategies become possible. These strategies are carefully discussed with clients, extending dialogue into action. Each strategy is sketched out by its creator, analyzed carefully by all to see if it does define the problem in accordance with the problematization, and then projected into an action format to determine if the people can assess potential risks and benefits.

7 Joining with clients in any action that advances their control over their own lives and that appears to be merited by the situation.

8 Learning to examine critically any actions as to process and outcomes.

The principles presented here underlie our concept of a social action strategy. They are not meant to represent a mechanistic formula for every situation, but rather are presented as practice principles we believe to be essential to any advocacy/empowerment practice, whatever the particular setting may be. Critical reflection and evaluation of action is an essential ingredient in this framework since the practice does not predetermine people's problems and roles. The commitment to critical reflection arises as a necessity to ensure the process of struggle to respond to the concrete issues in people's lives. The process is not an easy one, particularly when so many variables (income, housing, medication, etc.) are out of the control of the people and the staff of the program. The uncertainty/opportunity contradiction which we propose can lead people to desire a more structured, repetitive, assured environment when confronted continuously by the difficulty of the work. But, obviously, a liberating theory applies to staff as well as clients, and every effort must be made to support staff in their work. Solidarity, engagement in agency decision making, time for staff support systems to function, all reflect and produce the practice principles which staff are directed to create in their work with clients. These vehicles for support are valued as a basis for self-criticism and reflection of program processes in a context where oppression prevails. The commitment is to the process of transformation, not to winning any particular event in the struggle. Where critical reflection cannot provide information about how to fight in every situation, it may be able to identify other action arenas where the struggle can be pursued.

We turn now to those other arenas for a discussion of legal advocacy and organizing, program evaluation, and community organization. In each of the following chapters we attempt to demonstrate the use of the same practice principles described here. In this effort, we hope to encourage the development of a comprehensive scope for problem analysis and action.

CHAPTER 6

Legal Advocacy and Organizing

Practice which emphasizes the relation between objective conditions and subjective perception and experience cannot separate direct practice and its focus on empowerment from indirect forms of practice and their focus on advocacy. It would be partially correct to say that empowerment often leads to 'case advocacy,' while the larger frame of reference for advocacy might be called 'issue advocacy.' What makes this perspective only partially accurate is that it does not necessarily presume that there is an ongoing relationship between the two realms of problem definition and social action. We do make this assumption about the internal relatedness of both people and issues, but we separate the realms of activity on the basis of strategic choices. In every 'case-advocacy' matter there are vital issues, but none which can supersede the person whose life and courage have brought the particular issue forward at that moment in time. Yet, the issues represented by that person, and crystallized in the lives of the other people who share common oppression, must be addressed. Furthermore, when these issues are addressed, in the form of 'issue advocacy,' they cannot be severed from the lives of the people who were the primary reason for the emergence of the issue. Issues emerge from the lives of the people and must be represented to them throughout any process of advocacy which does not include them directly in the advocacy activities undertaken.

This chapter will discuss the advocacy activities of legal and legislative research, training, preparation and delivery of testimony before legislative and administrative bodies, preparation of legislative recommendations and constituency organizing for promotion or obstruction of particular pieces of legislation at the county and state levels.

We would like to refer to the chart which we used in Chapter 4 (see p. 81) as a reminder of the complexity of former patients' lives in relation to operating agencies and bureaucracies. This chart illustrates how crucial life issues that relate to income, housing, health and mental health services, and meaningful activities all revolve around one or many formal organizations that are legitimated to provide services by different levels of political jurisdiction. These agencies have different legislative authorizations, operating charters, policies and guidelines, rules and regulations, practices and personnel. Sophisticated organizational theory converges with personal experience to suggest that workers operating in any one of these agencies know relatively little about the foundation, procedural operations, legal base and grievance mechanisms of all other organizations which have impact on their clients' lives. This lack of knowledge does not reflect areas of specialization so much as it demonstrates an incoherent division of labor and its accompanying narrowness of vision when defining problems confronted by clients.

Because the multiplicity of agencies does exert tremendous influence on the daily life and well-being of all former patients (except perhaps the very wealthy few), and contours so much of what occurs, it is our responsibility to know how each of these organizations functions, what the full array of available legal rights and entitlements is and, where necessary, how to fight to challenge agency-based definitions of need and resource allocation.

When an advocacy/empowerment orientation to problem definition is the overriding conceptual framework (see Chapter 1), discussion with clients is often enhanced by readily available information about what the resource and/or legal issues are. From a basic descriptive presentation of social needs, for income, better housing, or health care, for example, the identification of responsible agencies is a relatively simple task. Far more difficult is the necessary chore of ferreting out the contradictions between authorizing legislation, policy guidelines, regulations and/or local office interpretations of functional responsibilities by operating agencies. One only has to go to a public welfare office as an applicant for any service to experience the difference between legislative intent, on the one hand, and experienced reality on the other. Consequently, at an early date in any program which has a commitment to an advocacy/empowerment approach to practice, research must be undertaken to identify the legislative foundations and intentions* for all relevant agencies. This process will include the laws which legitimate and authorize particular programs and benefits, the guidelines and operational procedures governing agency practices, and grievance mechanisms. While this is a rather large undertaking, it is nonetheless essential for an adequate advocacy/empowerment practice.

Utilization of resources to produce the information needed can be an insurmountable problem for agencies operating under contracts which measure units of service delivered as a basis for reimbursement, or for direct service agencies which are short-staffed and overworked. These operational facts of life do not serve as legitimate rationalizations for avoiding the responsibilities for gathering and synthesizing materials. It can be argued that the background research and language translation (from 'legal-ese') tasks or functions constitute units of 'indirect' service or even ancilliary contact. Where necessary, other avenues for producing the material can be located. Retired senior citizens' groups often have lawyers or other legally sophisticated people who can assume some of the background research responsibility. They can also be educated about the needs and interests of the ex-patient population along the way. Law schools are often looking for 'clinical' training experiences for their students and might be amenable to involvement with these issues; legal services agencies may have the inclination to do the work since they already have a great deal of the necessary information and can expand their client pool by participating and developing referral linkages; Schools of Social Work are required to produce field placements for students, and development of a 'legal advocacy' unit to do the research and analysis might be mutually useful; and other colleges and universities are eager to find 'internship' experiences for students capable of using their resources to produce the data required. It is necessary, however, for at least one staff person to serve as liaison to the people doing the investigative research to do quality assurance. This is necessary to make certain that the results of the inquiry distinguish between actual written, formal statements of law, regulations or guidelines and the idiosyncracies of conventional operating practices or local interpretations. Preliminary

---

* State and federal legislative agencies can often provide information on the history of any bill including the fate of earlier drafts or related legislation. This is valuable resource material for strategy development as it can identify sources of support and opposition within each house of the legislature as well as specify where in the legislative process obstacles are likely to occur.

drafts of interpretations of legal material must then be referred to public interest lawyers to make sure that accurate interpretations are being made. We find that legal services attorneys and/or their research resources are extremely valuable allies in this undertaking. (The Mental Health Law Project, 2021 L Street, N.W., Suite 800, Washington, D.C. 20036 (202–467–5730) is an excellent resource.) Working with local legal services agencies also establishes a more firm basis for mutual referrals of clients and a shared understanding of the empowerment aspect of the practice (see Chapter 4).

The process of legal investigation can be converted into empowerment activities that characterize day programs (see Chapter 5). Staff responsible for the day program can introduce the legislative or legal researchers at a community meeting. The staff present the legal researchers' function as a project-authorized activity that came about as a result of the critical commentary that program participants have shared. Reminders of the types of issues and the people who raised them can be represented together with an analysis of why legislative research or rights and entitlements research is being done. Since the issues which have emerged come from and reflect on the lives of the people, and act back directly on them, clients can be invited to participate in a group which provides feedback and 'language instruction' to the research team. Where appropriate, clients can also join the research team.

Participants become a formal group led by program staff. The group is convened each time the research people have produced or uncovered some useful material. The information is presented to the group, discussed as to its meaning and relevance in their lives, and returned to the researchers who have gained some understanding of how pertinent issues or legal violations express themselves in daily life. They have also learned what level of language must be used in writing a report on their findings. The information describing daily life experience related to the legal or legislative matter at hand then re-emerges in the form of examples in the draft of the written statement articulating the material or in supporting position papers. This draft is represented to the group who review it for accuracy in relation to the examples (and see the significance of their input) and for comprehension in relation to the language and legal-political point being illustrated. The process utilized recreates the social action strategy of elaboration-thematization-problematization-action/potentials discussed above (see Chapters 4 and 5).

An example of a statement of legal rights and entitlements prepared for ex-patients can be found in Appendix II. It was created through the process described above. The specific content of the material cannot be applied uniformly because many of the laws and policies are determined by specific state or county governments and are also subject to change over time. This material, in booklet form, has become a regular part of direct practice in both our day program component and in case management. They return information to the people previously elicited from them, but filtered through both a critical framework and an empowering process (see Taichman *et al.*, 1980a and 1980b).

The connection between subjective perception and feelings, elevated to social criticism through an empowerment-oriented practice, transformed into objective issues, and reformulated into useful resource material for the people, illustrates the advocacy/empowerment relationship as well as the interaction of direct and indirect forms of practice. The booklet becomes a part of the reality that is shared within the program. Its issues reflect mental patient's complaints transformed into political expressions; its language connotes citizenship rather than illness; its direction suggests action rather than acquiescence; and its framework posits adversarial rather than treatment relations with power holders. The booklets, therefore, are an invaluable 'tool' in direct practice in both empowerment processes and advocacy activities.

Other avenues for using advocacy emerge from whatever particular issue is created. When the value of the legal rights and entitlements material became obvious, and reflected itself throughout our direct practice activities, the potential for influencing other service providers arose. A grant proposal to publish the booklets and to provide advocacy-oriented training was prepared and funded through a local foundation (Veatch Program, North Shore Unitarian Church, Plandome, New York). Booklets containing the legal rights and entitlements material were published in readable language, an attorney was hired and free training was offered to mental health and social services workers responsible for after-care services. The training was divided into three segments, each half a day long, and agencies were offered the option of having the training on three consecutive half-days or one half-day of three consecutive weeks. The booklets were referred to the State Department of Social Services for review of the interpretations made of the law or the regulations under their jurisdiction and an enclosure was attached to each booklet identifying several points disputed by that agency with their verbatim comments included. Invitations were sent out to every agency, state hospital, mental health clinic, or after-care program in the broad geographic area where we are located. Telephone conversations were held with the appropriate administrators of the larger agencies (three state psychiatric hospitals) specifically to invite them and ask that they assist us with logistics by providing rooms for training sessions and sending proper notification to staff who might attend. Agency administrators were told by letter and telephone that the three sessions would cover a general introduction or orientation to legal issues in after-care, the specifics of the material included in the booklets and a general discussion about introducing the material to clients. Workers who attended the training sessions were told that the attorney doing the training and an experienced social worker would be available to them by telephone for follow-up consultation and/or clarification about how to use the booklets or on how to develop legal issues that arose in their practice.

Since all service providers with whom we were familiar operated out of a psychiatric or psycho-social orientation, the prospect of introducing legal advocacy materials was intriguing. From the start, scepticism about outcome was substantial. But, since one desired outcome was problem-posing to the agencies and their workers through teaching content that focused on clients' real needs, the process itself was seen as an advocacy activity. Indeed, the process proved interesting: the most common responses of workers to the first training session were very positive, and countless examples of legal abuses by homeowners and landlords were brought up by many people in each training cycle. By the second session, when several new trainees arrived (who were almost always supervisors), the enthusiasm had waned and was replaced by a barrage of hostile questions, often competitive in their antagonism. Workers demanded to know how this material could be useful to mentally ill people. Trainees asserted that it was futile to introduce legal issues to people who were frail, confused and vulnerable. They even talked about how legal thinking could produce 'decompensation.' We soon learned that these assaults were committed by workers whose supervisors attended the second or third training sessions or who were attacked at their place of work by supervisors who had been told about the workers' overt enthusiasm for the advocacy content by other workers participating in the training.

Ironically, the individual evaluations of the experience written by the trainees were predominantly positive.

The experience informed us that the ideological commitment to a medicalized model of mental health was firmly in place among the agencies that made up the local inter-organizational field or network of community-based service providers. This was obvious in our catchment area, where we had been under attack from the day our contract with the State Office of Mental Health had been announced. But, given the proliferation of rhetoric about community-based mental health services and the need for advocacy on behalf of former patients, the degree and especially the intensity of agency opposition to any information about legal rights and entitlements was a small surprise. It did poiny out an ironic situation: advocacy was overwhelmingly perceived to be an activity that was needed to get former patients orchestrated into patterns of consumption of pre-existing services that were developed around an orientation to problem definition which was contradictory to the clients' real needs. It was advocacy to meet agency needs concealed as clients' needs. This also expressed itself in calls from workers who wanted to know how to do 'case advocacy' in relation to issues which the owners of adult homes or SROs had brought to their attention – usually a problem with a missing SSI cheque or Medicaid card. The owners were clearly in control of the content of services as well as 'advocacy' and workers from agencies that participated in mental health 'teams' which included homeowners or managers clamored to get information about advocacy that served their 'team' members' interests. Thus, in the distorted world of mental health practice, case managers and other workers demanded to know advocacy practices which served the interests of their clients' foremost oppressors. When the real interests of their clients were separated from the interests of the profit sector homeowners or facility managers, there were no inquiries or issues raised.

The combination of workers' initial enthusiasm and overt agency censorship indicated that we needed to escalate the issue of agency compliance to dysfunctional models of community-based care. The decision to pose the inter-organizational field as an ideological problem was converted into a strategy based on evaluation of our training efforts. Rather than simply using the conventional pre-test/post-test attitudinal scale to measure what people felt about the training (we already had positive post-training data), we decided to assess the communications system within agencies to explore the way organizational structure and/or ideology functioned to enhance or to obstruct new perspectives on practice. Using our freely provided training as the focus of investigation, interviews were conducted with workers and supervisory personnel in each agency to whom training was provided. We wanted to know about the actual utilization of the legal advocacy materials, not about how workers felt about the training experience. Since practice is the only valid test of educational efforts, the outcome would be a simultaneous assessment of our training and its interface with an antagonistic ideology.

After approximately eighty individuals were interviewed, systematic patterns appeared with undeniable regularity. Only one worker who received the legal advocacy training was using it as a framework and using the legal rights and entitlements booklets with clients. This individual was doing so without authorization from her unit chief, as she presumed that permission to attend the training sessions was tantamount to permission to use the content learned. Since she was located in a community-based clinic attached to a catchment area unit of a state hospital, her unit chief never knew what she was doing as the unit chief never went out into the community. When the unit chief learned that this worker was using the legal advocacy material, he stopped it immediately (Johnson *et al.*, 1982).

All of the other workers who had received training also clearly received one message, however it may have been issued: the material was irrelevant, dangerous to clients and potentially threatening to any worker or program. The lack of pertinent meaning derived from the fact that the agencies' definition of problems facing former patients was medical-psychiatric in nature. It was confined to such issues as medication maintenance, attending mental health clinics and going to other similarly construed rehabilitative programs. The legal rights material was presumed to be 'dangerous' to clients in that it could produce either 'decompensation' or eviction from the placement. And it was ominous for workers or programs because anyone carrying around such information as could be found in the rights and entitlements booklets was bound to be thrown out of the adult homes or SROs by the management or owners.

Homeowner control over the internal relations of conventional agency operated programs was demonstrated. Agencies cooperating in 'treatment teams' with owners or managers were shown to be engaged in conflicts of interest and collusion. Fear of owners emerged as the guiding hand rationalizing justification of support for domination and exploitation through medicalized definitions of ex-patients' problems (Johnson *et al.*, 1982).

Any time an agency, program or community organization attempts to produce change in its domain or in its practice, there invariably follows an educational or training program. When the change is approved by the hierarchy in a larger scale organization, e.g., a State Office of Mental Health in relation to its component parts at the service delivery level, a series of assumptions about the change occur. It is presumed to have a self-evident rationality, to be compatible either instantly or reasonably quickly with previous modes of practice, thought and/or workers' identity. And it is presumed to be dissemi-nated through the organizational system coherently and integrated equally in all operating units. As indicated in the Introduction to this book, systems planners and administrators are as capable of arbitrarily declaring rationality to be pervasive among their staff as that same staff is capable of perceiving irrationality among their clients. The local inter-organizational field, committed over time to an institutional model of mental health care and to the prerequisite model of disabled patients, cannot easily accommodate transformations. When genera-tions of worker identity and professional reinforcement through train-ing and association retain outmoded practices, resistance within bureaucracy must be expected. Our research demonstrates the recal-citrance of the old guard and its model of care as well as their resilience in the face of new federal initiatives and changes in state mental health policy. It also demonstrates what occurs when change within a system, from an institutional model to a community-based system of care, is seen by administrators as only a technical or administrative problem rather than a political or ideological confrontation. And it demons-trates that significant change within a large organization requires a conflict-oriented strategy to accomplish its objectives rather than a more obfuscatingly rationalized cooperative model.

The learning gained from the training/evaluating process confirmed two realities: SRO residents had virtually no protection from exploita-tion or arbitrary control by owners or managers of the places where they lived, and adult home residents, who had ample legislative and regulatory protection, were in fact obstructed from having their rights protected by a regulatory agency that operated from a pro-owner bias. Time after time the regulatory agency refused to challenge homeow-ners' right to evict case managers, whole programs or residents. After every effort to negotiate a possible way to guarantee access of workers to their clients in adult homes failed, and an untested presumption of the primacy of private property rights over human civil rights was assumed by the regulatory agency, a new strategy had to be sought. The same conclusion was reached after struggling to identify a workable approach to the SRO landlords' tyranny.

A significant part of the problem that arose within both the adult homes and the SROs occurred because using legal recourse required that residents of the homes (the clients of our programs as well as other service providers such as mental health clinics) become the active plaintiffs in any legal case. Legal services agencies could not justify having an agency as a client and other available legal resources could not adequately explain how an agency that is denied access to its clients could conceivably meet the test of an injured party. They could easily see how a client denied access to his/her worker or prevented from expressing his/her choice of program could be viewed as so injured. Any analysis of former patients' lives in adult homes or SROs informs those familiar with the situation that any resident who takes part in a lawsuit against an owner that was a member of a 'treatment team' including staff from the state hospital mental health clinic, was very likely to be rehospitalized. This threat, used or implied, against frail and highly vulnerable people, quite successfully obstructs much of the deserved participation in or follow-through with client-initiated lawsuits. The regulatory agency is freed from responsibility by invoking an individual defect model explanation: if the residents really felt intimidated, as we claimed they did, then they were free to make complaints about owners to the regulatory agency or to file a legal grievance. (It is not atypical for a regulatory or code enforcement agency to call an owner or a mental health clinic to check on a complainant's 'reliability.') The regulatory agency and other mental health agencies claimed the fact that the ex-patients would not step forward to file legal complaints indicates how 'misguided advocacy' could become distorted and 'biased' against the owners or other 'team' members.

Trying to rally support for a fight against profit-sector owners by agencies in the inter-organizational network will prove useless in relation to those agencies using a medicalized view of problems and therapies. They perceive their own organizational and professional interests to be synonymous with the interests of their clients, as we pointed out in the data related to advocacy training. The responses of mental health agencies using medicalized problem definitions were heightened in their absurdity. Problems posed to homeowners by advocacy-oriented programs or fully justified lawsuits brought by a resident of a home were seen as cutting back on available beds for discharge of present inpatients. Holding patients in the hospital when they no longer needed that level of care was against their constitutional right to treatment in the least restricted setting. Discharging people into homes characterized by domination and exploitation, however, and allowing homeowners to use fear of eviction of workers or residents as their control over state-funded after-care programs (by controlling the content of case management, for example, so that it never dealt with issues related to the conditions in the home) was not seen as a problem.

Agencies most centrally involved with the quality of life of former patients were useless in any political mobilization to protect clients' rights or to assure their entitlements to written legislative guarantees spelled out in the law. The advocacy struggle, like the community organization struggle discussed in Chapter 8, had to extend beyond the ideological and inter-organizational network of service providers whose interpretation of functional responsibilities constituted a betrayal of the interests of former patients in favor of the profit interests of homeowners and the professional interests of mental health agencies.

The issue approached first was related to the lives of former patients residing in SROs. This type of housing includes everything from a rooming house with four or more people (in New York) all the way up to the 'welfare hotel,' which could house as many as several hundred. Conditions in these places, particularly the profit-operated hotels, are often abominable; residents are often as safe as their physical strength. The populations include frail elderly, former patients of state hospitals, parolees from jails and prisons, alcoholics and drug abusers, and other poor people unable to locate decent housing. No federal or New York state law offered protection. Clients bring stories of physical abuse and rape, of being given arbitrary rent figures and of being denied SSI personal allowance money, of filth and horrible food, and of frequent arbitrary eviction. Homeless people have described the streets as a safer environment. It was not uncommon for a landlord to move people arbitrarily and precipitiously from one SRO residence to another in a different neighborhood or community without the person's permission or prior knowledge.

Efforts to address this problem came from direct practice. In case management and through the day program we attempted to organize a residents' council in an SRO hotel. This followed months of complaints by clients, active involvement of a civil association in support of residents, and continual efforts to follow every issue carefully. A community monitoring system was set up. Members of the civic association, invited by our program to attend negotiating meetings with the landlord, were invited by residents to visit in the SRO. The visit was the premise for monitoring changes that were promised by the landlord. Discrepancies were raised by local community civic leaders rather than by vulnerable clients/residents or by our project which would have been accused of being anti-landlord. When this method proved successful, but limited, a joint committee of staff and community people decided to move in the direction of formulating a 'Rental Agreement.' This was an effort to take many of the rights and entitlements existing in landlord-tenant law and apply this body of law to SRO landlords and their renters who were former patients. The Rental Agreement generated controversy in the inter-organizational system as hospital staff and mental health agency administrators were reluctant to cooperate, again because they thought that landlords would refuse to participate, and would thus decrease available beds for future discharges.

Clearly, promoting legal rights and entitlements for former patients will not come about through mental health system policy or practice so long as that system is medicalized in its thought structure and systems-rationality-oriented in its strategy. Agencies at the local service delivery system level, whether operational units of state hospitals or voluntary sector agencies under contract to provide mental health service, will not provoke conflict with landlords when there is any risk to the agency's concept of its own self-interest, regardless of the harm it may cause to their clients. Constituency building for change must come from outside associations whose interests can be coalesced for either short or long term alliance. And the vehicle for producing change must be outside the domain controlled by the system which is the target of an advocacy effort: that is, it must be outside the administrative control of a bureaucracy, at least in the beginning.

Development of legislation can be a strategically significant arena for advocacy practice. When it became apparent that few organizations within the service delivery system would actively campaign for residents of SROs to have the same protection and rights which exist for all other tenants, the relevant action arena shifted to the legal-legislative realm. After a survey of legislative authorities to identify state legislators with historically demonstrated concerns for ex-patients, SRO residents or tenants, a series of discussions was initiated to identify potential sources for sponsoring project-initiated legislation. Rather than trying to create a new piece of mental health or social services law, it became apparent that the most significant change could be brought about by seeing the problem generically, in landlord-tenant terms. A bill was drafted that amended existing legislation to include SRO residents in the basic set of rights and protections which already exist in Landlord-Tenant law. A copy of the final bill is included as Appendix III along with samples from a brochure (Appendix II). These materials explain the bill to mental health and legal services agencies and suggest how the bill might be used with clients. Accompanying the more technical information is a strategy which addresses how the new legislation might be converted into action projects to protect former patients and other SRO residents and how it might be incorporated into direct service programs as a process of empowerment.

Once freed from trying to enlist allies among disinterested agencies, very positive prospects for coalitions emerge. Among potential allies there are legal services agencies, civil liberties groups (if you can prove or suggest discrimination), some religious organizations interested in progressive social programs, organizations of the elderly ranging from the Grey Panthers to lesser known advocacy organizations, and associations or advocacy groups whose primary constituency is made up of people who are forced to rely upon SRO housing. In addition, housing groups and tenants' associations can be involved because the legislative arena and the issues raised have been part of their turf for many years. Organizing these groups in support of a particular bill produces an ironic outcome: from virtual non-existence as a legislative entity at the start, anyone with a letterhead and a competent organizing strategy can appear to be a knowledgeable and potentially powerful lobby. Writing letters explaining the issues, developing a position paper to provide a context and rationale, and arguing the merits of a particular bill and why it is the preferred alternative (see Appendix IV for an example of such a package) communicates to legislators, their staff people and potential allies that one knows how to operate in the legislative arena. These activities also function effectively to convince legislators either to sponsor or to co-sponsor a bill, a crucial support step in the eventual struggle for passage.

Relations with legislators' key staff people, particularly legislative assistants to sponsors or co-sponsors of a bill and staff members of legislative committees, are central to advocacy efforts in legislative strategies. These people very often are thoroughly knowledgeable about the formal and informal processes and procedures of bill passage. They know about personality obstacles among legislators or staff that may slow down or obstruct movement through committees, and about interventions from competing lobbying groups attempting to reach other legislators. These resourceful people can also inform a coalition of efforts being made by those opposed to a bill to kill it or modify its wording so that lead time for mobilizing a telephone, telegram and/or letter writing campaign can be mounted to preserve the legislation or the internal integrity of a bill. Equally important is identification of people within the coalition or alliance whose networks of support are extensive and/or influential so that these people can be quickly summoned to step in and support the bill when or if it comes under attack. Keeping these strategically important people updated on every step of the process is required to maintain discipline sufficient to respond rapidly to the vagaries or dynamics of political activity in the legislative process.

Having been successful in the Landlord-Tenant arena, and securing passage guaranteeing SRO residents all of the rights of tenants, the task shifts to informing service providers and others who might benefit from the legislation. Since most agencies and/or individuals whose interests might be served by this legislation will not automatically be informed about it, or necessarily see the connection between it and clients to whom it might apply (see earlier material on medicalization in Chapter 1), a notification sheet and guide were prepared and mailed to all known after-care and legal services programs in the state (Appendix III). In addition to describing the bill and its potential use, other legal advocacy materials are mentioned and made available upon request. Any requests that do come in alert us to another potential ally for future legislative struggles.

The next issue forced into a legislative arena involved adult homeowners' apparent power to control who was entitled to have access to the residents of their licensed and regulated facilities. Involuntary evictions of an entire program staff from two adult homes, failure to find support from the regulatory agency, and an unwillingness to act aggressively outside common domain boundaries by the Office of Mental Health all coincided to lead to an attempt to identify potential sponsors in the state legislature for a new bill on access. A survey of related legislation was conducted across the nation and progressive legislation reviewed for proper wording to accomplish the objective of having the right of access to residents transcend the private property right of landlords. The prominent issues involve who would determine who would be allowed in the building and under what circumstances. As with the first legislative effort, a position paper is prepared together with a draft of suggested legislation (see Appendix V). Legislators and legislative staff people previously known to us are contacted by phone, informed of the issue and asked to provide advice on potential sponsors in both houses of the legislature. Position papers and draft legislation are circulated, comments solicited and refinements made until action sponsors are identified. The process from that point on follows the same one outlined above. In this case, however, one significant difference did emerge – very powerful opposition, in the form of the adult homeowners' lobby, made its impact known. As a result, we are able to expand our knowledge of advocacy and organizing in the legislative arena.

Advocacy efforts in the legislature are dependent upon successful communication and positive alliances. Communication often becomes a moment to moment phenomenon: sponsors', co-sponsors' and legislative staff members' commitments and understandings are not necessarily exactly the same as the advocacy group responsible for developing the legislation. Legislators and their staff engage in negotiations with opposing constituencies, such as the homeowners' lobby, without always realizing the full significance of all of the stipulations or particular language in a given bill. As a result, they may inadvertently trade off some passage or wording that is central to the purpose of the bill without recognizing the impact of their proposed compromises. Consequently, once any known opposition emerges, regular contact with key legislative staff working on the bill must be maintained, members of the support network must be alerted to prepare a rapid response, and constituencies within the legislature must be contacted to develop a workable strategy to try to offset opposing interests. Our experience is that a sophisticated, powerful lobbyist can quietly negate or terminate a bill that is less than a high priority issue for the sponsors (as is frequently the situation with advocacy legislation). This tactic works far more effectively in a state where each House in the legislature is controlled by a different political party. An example in the case of the access bill occurred at one point where wording so dramatically different was inserted into one of the sponsor's versions that an interim strategy had to be developed as a fallback position to have the bill killed because of the newly proposed wording. Similar 'behind the scenes' input into legislative developments occur after passage by one or both houses of the legislature or while the approved bill awaits the signature of the governor. Similar response patterns, based on constant communication with legislative supporters and their staff, have to be prepared for saturation of the Governor's Office by constituencies in favor of the bill.

Monitoring legislative developments and the ways in which powerful lobby groups subtly as well as overtly influence legislation suggests another arena for advocacy efforts – intervention into processes and procedures for developing guidelines and regulations are constantly brought before legislative committees and administrative public hearings (see Appendix V for an example of a position paper developed to contend against proposed revisions in adult home regulations. Rather than include any specific information here, we have just reprinted the preamble as an illustration of problem redefinition at the policy level).

Committees of the legislature meet routinely in open hearing to take public testimony; sub-committees of the legislature often do the same, but with less formal notice. Ad hoc sub-committees of any legislative standing committees can often be created, usually by members of the majority party, to undertake exploration or examination of a specific issue. This avenue is often one possibility that can lead to broad public exposure and later action on some controversial issues that a regular standing committee might not pursue. Similarly, the operating agencies of state or city governments hold public hearings to invite or accept comments on major revisions of their regulations, an act often required by law. In all of these settings, actions are proposed and often taken which impact on the lives of former patients. Positive relationships with legislative people can provide information to advocacy groups about which committees and agencies are holding hearings, about where the hearings will be located and what issues will be salient.

Advance notice of meetings of legislative committees or agency hearings on regulations provide a potential forum for advocacy positions to be advanced in public. Introduction of advocacy organizations' positions must be strategically examined in relation to whether the issue at hand is one where ideological disparity exists in obvious form. Where conflict can be anticipated, an approach must be developed to cultivate a constituency among potential legislative supporters that are not tied to conventional mental health system paradigms of theory or practice. Because the agencies historically legitimated by the state know when hearings are held that could impact on their domains, they and their supporters (e.g., contract agencies) regularly attend these hearings to present testimony. Staff from legislative committees and sub-committees often use the combination of prepared written testimony and tape recordings (later converted into typed transcriptions) of oral testimony and dialogue to prepare legislative recommendations. Where conventional agencies and their supporters are the only sources of information or input for final reports and recommendations, the outcome of the hearings is typically controlled by one conceptual frame of reference.

Participation in written submissions and oral delivery of testimony at every available opportunity, whether at a legislative or administrative hearing, is a vital area of advocacy activity. Contributions of a written and oral form that articulate an alternative framework for examining issues, and which can critically expose the drawbacks of conventional mental health policy and practice, can have significant impact on policy-makers in legislative positions. Position papers and presentations at hearings also serve as important sources of contact within legislative committees. Anticipating 'command performances' by mental health providers from state agencies and other parts of the service delivery system, and projecting what their positions will be, provide a context for advocacy representation. Taking care to ensure that the most powerful agencies and individuals speak first (e.g., the Commissioner of Mental Health, or a representative from that office), the advocacy position includes criticism of the major agencies' input into the formal record as part of the testimony. Written material is always included, but not read verbatim. Oral testimony expands issues raised in the written material (copies of which are presented to all committee members), doubling the input into the resource base or formal record of the hearing from which legislative staff prepare recommendations. Opposition points of view or postures on particular issues are critically assessed and related back to the issues raised in the written document. Questions raised as part of the testimony can be designed to produce interaction with committee members that furthers the validity and legitimacy of the advocacy orientation directly or enhances the critique of the opposition. Previous alliances with legislators or staff often produce questions prepared in advance to ask people representing different organizations and interests. It can also allow for access to drafts of committee reports for further pre-publication input.

Systematic, precisely worded and concisely argued positions, with non-rhetorical, non-inflammatory language, and useful, realizable recommendations have maximum influence. At the very least, they provide for a problem-posing data base that can be expanded or reintroduced at a more favorable time or in a more favorable place or context. Examples of testimony are included in the Appendix VI to demonstrate the presentation of our ideological position before a Congressional Sub-Committee as well as before state legislature committees.

Quite obviously, tying advocacy to the program base of empowerment in direct practice requires both the resources to devote to the advocacy arena and a commitment to the practice. The legislative examples presented above demonstrate how issues which develop or emerge in the context of direct practice escalate into another arena of activity. The legal rights and entitlements example demonstrates the process of returning to the people the information they provide. This information is then used in a different forum. The commitment to empowerment/advocacy as a framework requires action be continuous, mutually supportive and integrated between both sectors of concern. The issue, which will reappear as a dimension of our next chapter on program evaluation, is whether an advocacy/empowerment-oriented program, anchored by choice or contract to provision of direct services, can see its way clear to engage in the types of advocacy activities discussed here.

We prefer to see this issue as one influenced at least as much by ideological commitments as it is by strained resources. This point is stressed because a firm commitment to a conceptual framework similar to the one presented here removes the issue from the realm of choice. The critical question is one of resource allocation, of how to accomplish the array of activities suggested here, or created by staff, that do not get reimbursed under service provision commitments in grants or contracts. The problem is defined as an active confrontation rather than a passive, acquiescence to external demands, that it simply cannot be done because of budget constraints. The time required to produce many of the advocacy activities discussed above can be dramatically reduced when the process of network or constituency building is presumed to be a prerequisite to sustained functioning. Community connections, discussed below in Chapter 8, are clearly required for simple survival as well as for development; legislative connections have a similar function for development and legitimation.

The time and staff resources usually assumed necessary to coordinate agency activity with other service providers frequently amount to a waste of time for an advocacy/empowerment-oriented program. The vast gulf and meaning of ideological disparity has already been discussed at length. It suggests that time and energy committed to efforts to rationalize and coordinate services across ideological chasms is time and energy discarded (to be sure, we do not dismiss proforma attendance at selected meetings, or attendance useful to information gathering). Meeting with those actual or potential individuals and groups with whom one can develop common interests, or in building strategic alliances, can replace the more typical and useless meetings seemingly incumbent upon many administrative and supervisory staff. Once the positive relationships and communications systems are in place, the amount of time necessary to devote to gather the information discussed above, or to prepare the materials for presentation, decreases substantially. One becomes part of a network and privy to its information flow as well as a contributor to its content and development. Other, longer range plans involving building closer community ties and involving community people can be envisioned as well. The salient issue is commitment to the principles of the advocacy/empowerment paradigm. The residual problem is its strategic implementation. Similar concerns will be obvious as we turn to program evaluation, a multi-faceted process of inestimable value, but usually thought to be a luxury at best, or an obstacle to be endured.

CHAPTER 7

Program Evaluation

The importance of setting aside staff time and designating responsibility for program evaluation in a program utilizing an advocacy/empowerment approach cannot be underestimated. Often, where resources are stretched, arrangements can be made with universities to provide internships, etc., as a vehicle for offsetting costs; however, the research must be under control of the program with regard to instrument design, data collection process, and publication. Obviously, the person responsible for the program evaluation *must* share the advocacy/empowerment perspective. An appropriately conceived program evaluation can help sustain program direction and guidance through providing critical reflection; it can create systematic, data-based responses that enhance program survival in a turbulent and hostile environment; it can contribute to building working agenda for staff and clients in case management and/or day programs and it can create assertive strategies in the program's struggle to advocate for social change. In this chapter, we will explore several questions or issues regarding the purposes, pitfalls, designs, methodologies, tools and uses of advocacy/empowerment program evaluation. Here are a number of concerns which occurred to us over time:

- Why should a community-based, advocacy/empowerment-oriented agency engage in program evaluation?
- Can we directly infuse evaluative data into the program?
- Can the process itself be useful to the respondents?
- How can we justify the commitment of scarce resources?
- How does this type of evaluation differ from other types?

– What are the pitfalls of partial and inadequate approaches to program evaluation?
– Can we conceptualize program evaluation consistently with our overall design?
– What should be included and excluded from its design?
– What sorts of research instruments might be effectively utilized?

We offer here some tentative and modest suggestions, based upon our experience, as to how these questions might usefully be pursued. We also discuss the specific purposes, design and methodology of a case example of our own Community Support System Project (CSSP).

Purposes of advocacy/empowerment evaluation

We had four purposes for program evaluation in our CSSP: (1) to help develop a process of critical reflection for both the program staff and clients; (2) to help create a defensive strategy against inter-organizational attack; (3) to help develop an assertive strategy to support our advocacy activities; and (4) to generate empirical data to elaborate and specify our theoretical understanding of the social change process within an inter-organizational field. These purposes derive from the awareness that rigorous, empirically-generated data are critical for the successful pursuit of the program's advocacy/empowerment goals, and for the maintenance of organizational survival (see Rose, *Betrayal of the Poor*, 1972 and Warren, Rose and Bergunder, *The Structure of Urban Reform*, 1974, for an elaboration of this assumption). The purposes also mirror the project's dual focus of client empowerment and inter-organizational advocacy by placing the concrete life situation of the client, and the project's inter-organizational dynamics, at the center of the evaluation.

Critical reflection – integration of theory and practice

The systematic interaction of theory and practice within a community-based human service organization is greatly facilitated by the institutionalization of a program evaluation component into the organization. Agencies that engage in various forms of direct practice with clients can become submerged in the mass of daily demands, details and rigors of practice and can lose sight of larger theoretical issues, or even agency objectives. The literature on organizations is replete with discussions of goal displacement and the subversion of organizational purposes by an organization's own maintenance needs. This 'activism' or non-reflective activity (Freire, 1973) or 'case-work mentality' (Mills, 1959) can obscure the social definition (see Chapter 1) of many human problems and eventually lead to a de facto reduction to the acceptance and practice of an individual defect model of causation and solution (Warren *et al.*, 1974). To the extent that this model ignores valid social causality or objective conditions, the action based upon it will be self-defeating – that is, socially constructed problems are reduced ('subjectivized') to individual defect problem definitions which require 'therapeutic' solutions that do not address the essential problems. The constant frustrations stemming from attempting solutions which do not address fundamental causes, in turn, often results in passivity, cynicism and 'burn-out' for both program staff and clients.

To help the organization avoid activism, to make the individual defect model programming and its impact itself a focus for critical investigation, and to move toward more soundly constructed, theoretically guided action, program evaluation must analyze the organization, not only in terms of how well it is doing what it is doing; it must also ask whether what the program is doing is the correct approach – i.e., is the program's problem definition and solution strategy the correct one in the first place. Reinhardt (1973) terms the first criterion (measuring how well it is doing what it is doing), the program's 'microquality' and the second (assessing whether what it does is correct), its 'macroquality' (Scott, 1981 and Pfeffer and Salancik, 1978 develop a similar distinction in their concepts of efficiency and effectiveness). To approach the macroquality question requires a broadening of the scope of analysis to include an evaluation of the action paradigm itself.

Macroquality analysis is especially important for advocacy/empowerment-oriented programs which challenge the problem definition prevalent in the institutionalized thought structure. Warren alerts us to this when he states that:

> The power to define the problem, or in our terms, to impose one's own diagnostic paradigm and its attendant institutionalized thought structure, is especially pertinent to the conducting of research. In considering the supportive role of social research, it is important to recognize that most of the prevalent research takes as its point of departure the prevalent diagnostic paradigm. (Warren, 1977, pp. 497–8)

Macroquality analysis avoids making the prevalent thought structure or dominant ideology its point of departure for development of instruments and data; instead, it makes the thought structures themselves foci of investigation.

Once the macroquality issues have been addressed, the microquality issues can be pursued; how effective is the program at doing what it does? Structural, process and outcome indicators can be utilized to determine effectiveness (Scott, 1977). For our CSS project, the critical microquality issue was how to translate the program's problem definition and practice principles into program evaluation practice (process and methods) that would provide relevant feedback to both staff and clients. How could the substance and process of our research parallel the advocacy/empowerment orientation of the project? How might its substance and process be used effectively to benefit clients/staff?

Since the project's orientation had a dual focus – advocacy at the inter-organizational level and empowerment at the client level – our evaluation had to analyze the program's interactions and effects on both of these levels. We developed a Social Profile interview questionnaire (see Appendix VII) to document the quality of life of the program's clients and the extent to which they were receiving their full range of rights and entitlements. Our quality of life indices included: community integration, quality of housing, quality of medical care, quality of mental health care, quality of after-care and social service programs. We also developed a data collection format to determine the frequency, nature and outcome of the program's inter-organizational interactions. The dual foci of our research will be discussed in more detail later in this chapter, but let it suffice here to say that the aggregated data provided an invaluable resource for an overview of problems and issues confronting the agency; guidance for both clients and the agency; agenda setting information and redirection; and a base for strategy formulation for the advocacy and inter-organizational activities of the project. The process also allowed clients another structured opportunity to reflect upon their full range of rights and entitlements, to assess what their current situation was in relation to recognizing and realizing legal guarantees, and to examine why they were not receiving what they needed.

Thus, advocacy/empowerment program evaluation can help emancipate a program from the 'trap of activity' and help rejuvenate burned-out program staff and clients by providing critical overviews and insights into the interaction between project purposes and daily practice. It thus serves the function of providing a critical representation to staff and clients of the progress they are making and the obstacles (if any) they are confronting. By seeing the myriad of personal problems as reflecting broader social and organizational issues, both staff and clients have a better understanding of their work and lives and, therefore, more control over them. It is in this sense that advocacy/empowerment program evaluation serves the purpose of critical reflectivity.

Defense against inter-organizational attack

Human service organizations utilizing the advocacy/empowerment approach by definition challenge the prevalent problem definitions and program practices within the inter-organizational field. They are subject to a hostile reaction from those organizations most committed to prevalent problem definitions and practice models. Advocacy/empowerment program evaluation can provide a very useful defensive or reactive function in helping the advocacy/empowerment program maintain organizational survival in the face of inter-organizational hostility. Systematic documentation by the CSSP staff of each instance of inter-organizational conflict can provide the basis upon which the conflicts can be focused on substantive issues rather than mired in ad hominem or personality attacks and innuendo. The strategy of documentation of conflicts and keeping all conflicts issue-centered and public has the effect of disarming attempts by hostile organizations within the inter-organizational field to either destroy or coopt the advocacy/empowerment program. It also provides a systematic data base to use in community constituency building activities (see Chapter 8). Thus, program survival as well as autonomy is enhanced.

Warren *et al.* (1974) have shown that a new organization entering an inter-organizational field can expect a certain amount of initial turf competition and conflict. These turf conflicts usually center around domain resources such as funding, personnel, clients or geographical areas of service. After some initial skirmishes, most inter-organizational interactions that continue are usually reduced to marginal boundary adjustments. However, if the new organization also has a challenging problem definition to the prevalent one – which, in the case of human service organizations, is an individual defect model – then an increase in the quantity and intensity of conflict can be expected. The very legitimacy of organizations (or unfettered access to its domain resources and activities) is the central issue of these paradigmatic conflicts, which accounts for their intensity. Thus, new advocacy/empowerment organizations should consider it probable that they will be met with some degree of serious, program-threatening conflict in their inter-organizational environment and prepare themselves for it.

Our CSSP was aware that the inter-organizational field it entered was dominated by medicalized psychiatric program models. One major strategy the CSSP adopted to cope with this set of dynamics was to utilize program evaluation to document in detail the nature of its inter-organizational interaction. The systematic, detailed recording and assessment of program contacts with all other organizations proved to be an invaluable resource for program policy guidance as well as a defense of the agency and its staff. The ability to produce concrete data showing the attacks of other agencies against the program to be substantively groundless, entirely self-serving and devoid of client-centered issues of proper care, and systematically obstructionist has the effect over time of reducing these types of attacks. This defensive strategy was a primary purpose for including program evaluation in the CSSP.

Assertive advocacy strategy for social change

The third purpose of our use of program evaluation was to generate supporting data in our efforts to advocate for change in the quality of life made available to our clients. Systematic data showing service gaps or deficiencies and the inability or unwillingness of organizations (both service providers and regulatory agencies) to provide their mandated services have proven to be a powerful weapon at the state legislative level, and at the state and regional offices of mental health. When the regular and structured inadequacies of the service delivery system are documented, the state is forced into a situation in which it either has to act to ameliorate the situation, or fail to act and reveal its rhetoric of comprehensive service delivery to be without substance. If the latter option of no action is chosen by the state, then the issues move from the technical realm of service delivery to the political realm of conflicts of interests. It is in this process of forcing the issue through documentation that the issues and support systems become clarified and the stage set for more effective advocacy strategies.

Generate empirical data – elaborate and specify for social change process

It has become clear, for example, that New York State's interest in integrating deinstitutionalized mental patients into the community and providing them with comprehensive services is mediated by its fiscal interest in maintaining a low inpatient population by discharging patients, often regardless of the settings. Our CSSP's documentation of the horrible living conditions in some housing, of the need for binding rental agreements guaranteeing tenants' rights, of the need for effective regulation, and for legislation insuring case manager access to Adult Homes has led to a series of actions to improve these conditions. However, at times, the project's actions have been met with resistance by the mental health and social service agencies. These interactions are also documented, often to provide a data base for pursuing legislative solutions to administrative obstacles (e.g., a bill to guarantee case managers access to their clients in private proprietary 'homes' offsets the failure of the state regulatory agency to fight for residents' rights). Documentation of organizational failures to function effectively from local to state levels (or within the 'vertical system') can also serve as an ongoing tool to bring community pressure to bear on legislative endeavors. Thus, the political and economic issues of after-care become salient with political mobilization as the necessary action strategy. It is in this manner that program evaluation can function as a data resource base for assertive advocacy. To change the objective conditions which contour the quality of daily life for ex-patients, our project's purposes for utilizing program evaluation for critical reflection for defense against inter-organizational attack and for assertive advocacy strategy make program evaluation a valuable investment for the advocacy/empowerment-oriented agency. However, the usefulness of program evaluation can be seriously impaired if the evaluator succumbs to a number of partial approaches to evaluation which have the effect of obscuring the distinction between the program's macroquality and its microquality. This obscurantism is accomplished by failing to include in the evaluation design crucial program effectiveness indicators such as the inter-organizational thought structure of the inter-organizational field, program outcomes and program implementation processes, which bring into focus the larger macroquality issues.

Each of the partial approaches to program evaluation research criticized in this chapter takes the prevalent institutionalized thought structure with its individual defect problem definition as its point of departure. By so doing, the resulting research findings serve to legitimate the existing institutionalized thought structure by removing it from critical focus. The validity of the findings are also suspect since to ignore, for instance, the effects of inter-organizational resistance on the implementation of outcome of a program can lead to erroneous conclusions regarding program success or failure.

Program evaluation research is of maximum value, we argue, when the advocacy/empowerment program's implementation, output, outcome and inter-organizational context are seen as internally related and centrally relevant for program success. With this comprehensive approach, policy and program planners are provided with a clear and valid understanding of what either facilitates or obstructs program success.

We now turn our discussion to the nature of these partial evaluation approaches followed by a discussion of our project's evaluation research design, methodologies and research tools.

Pitfalls of partial approaches to program evaluation

The evaluation approaches discussed below are partial to the extent that they fail to address important dimensions of a program, such as the intra-organizational and inter-organizational processes that have profound effects upon program effectiveness. The partial approaches discussed here are: (1) the output approach; (2) the outcome approach; and (3) the acontextual approach.

The output approach

This approach equates outputs of a program with its performance, outcomes or impact. It assumes that a program is a success or failure to the extent that it fulfills its contractual obligations for the production of units of service or outputs. Thus, if the program produces the appropriate quantity of output – e.g., X number of units of service per month, or number of patient visits per month, or number of cases handled, or number of days worked by staff, etc. – the program is considered to be in fulfillment of its objectives (Rossi *et al.*, 1979, p. 60; Nachimus, 1979, p. 3). This assumption is fallacious, however, since it completely ignores the question of program performance or impact. It tells little, if anything, of the program's definition of the problem, its quality of services, or of the effects, outcomes or impact of the program on the target population. It assumes output to be identical with impact which is a useful assumption for funding agencies or fiscal policy planners such as the Division of the Budget. Program evaluation which does not address the *performance* of a program, that is, the extent to which program output has achieved its stipulated goals, will not provide useful client-focused information for program planning or for the formulation of social or administrative policy designed to improve program validity.

Unfortunately, the output fallacy is a very prevalent approach to program evaluation at the federal, state and local levels. The case management program of New York State Office of Mental Health, Community Support Systems Program, designed to provide after-care services for deinstitutionalized mental patients, is evaluated in terms of the quantity of 'units of service' (one unit of direct service equals fifteen minutes of worker contact with the client), the number of case manager days worked per quarter year, and the amount of money spent by the program per quarter year or a quarterly cost-per-unit-of-service measure. This typically quantitative measure of output not only misses program impact or performance, but also ignores the qualitative aspects of the program: not just how much case management service was delivered, but toward what objectives and with how much movement must be addressed, if a useful evaluation is to be accomplished. Susan Steindorff recognizes that failure when she concludes for both the federally-funded Community Support Program and State Community Support Systems Programs that: 'While questions concerning the actual outcome and impact of these service delivery systems remain in the forefront of our consciousness, they currently remain basically unanswered' (Steindorff, 1979, p. 13).

The output approach also successfully removes the dynamics of the inter-organizational field from evaluative concern by assuming them as given. Failure to address critically the nature of the inter-organizational domain consensus and prevalent ideology serves to reproduce the existing arrangements, and also to ignore important causal factors determining program success or failure. For a program seeking to produce changes in service delivery patterns at the local level, as is the goal of the New York State Community Support Systems Program, to reproduce the existing inter-organizational patterns is a serious program failure. To avoid addressing this failure by the use of partial and inadequate evaluative methodology based upon output measures alone condemns policy-makers to repeated failures, or quantitative reassessments. It will not answer questions about program success or failure from the client or goal attainment perspective or explain either, thus rendering it a useless evaluative tool.

The outcome approach

This approach assumes that a social program is a success or failure to the extent that it fulfills its goals as stipulated by the researcher. It utilizes a rather mechanical, experimental research design, and thus ignores three important program dimensions: (1) the process of program goal change or emergence; (2) the process of program implementation; and (3) the inter-organizational dynamics that affect the goals and implementation strategies of the program. To the extent that these dimensions are overlooked, the findings generated by this approach may be fallacious or inappropriately biased.

The outcome approach typically utilizes the classic experimental design or 'quasi-experiment' (Campbell, 1969). After ascertaining the program 'goals' and 'operationalizing' them into 'measurable indices,' the researcher conducts a 'pre-test' before the program intervention at time A, and a 'post-test' at time B, after the program intervention. Variations of this method are used depending on the nature of the available 'control group.' The net outcome of the typical experimental design could be formulated as follows:

Net Outcome – Difference in scores on outcome measures at time A, before intervention, and time B, after intervention, for the experimental group.

Minus

Differences in scores on outcome measures at time A, before intervention, and time B, after intervention, for the control group.

Minus or Plus

Stochastic effects or chance fluctuations in the measurements. (Rossi *et al.*, 1979, p. 185)

Since truly randomized control groups are rarely available in any social program context, a 'quasi-experimental' design is most often used. This involves constructing a control group that is comparable to the target group in essential respects utilizing *non*randomized selection methods. The formula for the net outcome utilizing the quasi-experimental approach is:

Net Outcome = Outcome for target population

Minus

Outcome for constructed control group

Minus or Plus

Stochastic error.

Although the outcome fallacy approach is far superior to the output fallacy, it suffers three major shortcomings. First, it is blind to the process of emergent program goals which may divert the program in midstream away from the original goals as embodied in the research measures. This blindness is a result of a subsidiary fallacy – the goals fallacy – which proceeds on the assumption that clearly definable goals exist, that everyone involved understands and agrees upon them and pursues them, that they will remain unchanged throughout the research, and that the service is in fact related to them. To the extent that an emergent goal process occurs, the findings of the experimental outcome approach become increasingly irrelevant. It is not very helpful to be told that you are not achieving goals you no longer wish to achieve. Goal change is quite common for social programs, especially medium- and short-range goals, since it is often in the process of program implementation that problems, needs and alternative strategies become more clear. Many social programs also operate less mechanically than these measures require in order to respond to client contexts; e.g., a decrease in welfare cheques, a new restrictive policy in SSI recertification, etc., can occur totally outside the control of an agency whose clients are deeply affected by the policy that has non-measurable impact on agency performance. Outcome research typically does not have the capacity to comprehend the context in which programs function and which often contour their operations.

Second, the outcome approach ignores the *process* of implementation of the *social action* program. It fails to elaborate which aspects of the program are working well and which aspects are not. To be told that your program failed to achieve its stated goals does not inform you of why or how it failed, or how the program might become more effective. One aspect of the program may have worked brilliantly, while another functioned dismally. These different aspects of the program would cancel each other out in the experimental outcome approach and thus valuable information would be lost that might be used for critical feedback and planning. The only use for the experimental outcome measure of program success or failure is in the decision to continue or eliminate the program. It is of no use to program directors and staff in their attempts to make the program better. For this it is necessary to combine the experimental outcome study with a program implementation process study.

Third, the outcome approach, like the output approach, also removes the inter-organizational context from critical focus of the investigation to background assumptions. The extent to which program goals and implementation processes are determined or influenced by often powerful inter-organizational dynamics goes unmeasured, and thus these dynamics become uncontrolled extraneous confounding variables (Rossi *et al.*, 1979). Until these variables are controlled for, major causes of program evaluation must be complemented with a program implementation and inter-organizational analysis to achieve a comprehensive understanding of the program.

The acontextual approach

This approach assumes that an adequate evaluation of a social program can be accomplished without an analysis of the surrounding organizational and political economic context. The relationships of the program to other agencies and organizations are taken as given and the research focus is confined to either an intra-organizational analysis of the process of program implementation, and/or measuring program impact (Nachimas, 1979, p. 5). However, it has been shown that the 'inter-organizational field' in which a program functions very often has profound effects upon the program's process of development and ability to achieve its desired outcomes (Warren *et al.*, 1974).

The inter-organizational field becomes especially intrusive into the affairs of agency to the extent that a program is new and/or utilizes an alternative paradigm to define problems and to create practice strategies. To the extent that a program possesses either of these characteristics, it will be subject to a certain amount of inter-organizational conflict. If a program is new in the field, it can expect to engage in turf struggles with the other agencies in the community around such organizational domain issues as funding, personnel and/ or clients. If the program is wielding an alternative paradigm to the prevalent one in the inter-organizational field, in addition to the domain issues referred to above, it can expect ideological confrontations around practice and legitimation issues. If the agency or program is both new *and* working out of an alternative paradigm, the intensity of the expected conflict increases exponentially (Warren *et al.*, 1974). The effects of these struggles upon program implementation and impact cannot be ignored, particularly since the energy and resources committed to conflict-oriented activity come from the same people and input resources expected to deliver services.

None of the program evaluation methods discussed thus far contemplate a conflict-saturated, turbulent and/or hostile inter-organizational environment. Thus, they can entirely overlook the determinants of operational processes and/or program outcomes. A brief example may clarify this issue: case managers from an advocacy/empowerment-oriented agency are thrown out of a profit-run congregate care facility by the owner. The state regulating agency sides with the owner and neither the mental health clinic nor the Adult Protective Services agency intercede, since both operate out of the individual defect paradigm and assume their relationship with the owner to be a 'team' arrangement. Consequently, for a two month period, the case management program is deflated in its output and in its outcome during the period it was barred from client contact.

The historical and political economic context within which social agency programs operate is almost never addressed in program evaluation research, yet it may prove to be the single most important influence determining program direction, success or failure. For example, severe federal funding cuts for social programs and the substitution of block grants for categorical grants can result in serious funding shortages for social programs and renewed political struggle for existing funds in block grants. This struggle for a shortage of funds will have profound effects on the nature of inter-organizational relations and thus on the effectiveness of individual agencies. Minor turf skirmishes will be more serious and intense, and cooperation among agencies necessary to provide comprehensive services will be more difficult. These political economic considerations will negatively affect programs in their attempts to accomplish their goals.

The extent to which the other organizations in the inter-organizational field are either unwilling or unable to provide support services to an advocacy/empowerment program's client population can very well prove to be an insurmountable obstacle for the program. These inter-organizational effects thus cannot go unnoticed in a comprehensive program evaluation. They should be documented as they occur by the construction and maintenance of ongoing inter-organizational contact files. This information is invaluable not only for program planning and improvement, but also for program survival.

Thus, the output, outcome and acontextual approaches to evaluation are seriously limited in their value as a result of their narrowly circumscribed view of the organization. Is there a way to merge the strengths of these three options while avoiding their defects? The advocacy/empowerment evaluation design is an attempt at such a merger.

Advocacy/empowerment program evaluation

The key to successful advocacy/empowerment program evaluation is to be both theoretically and practically useful; that is, to conduct a comprehensive analysis of the effectiveness of the agency such that the outcome and process of the evaluation provides policy planning and critical learning functions for agency staff and clients. To accomplish both of these goals, it is necessary to capture the structural and processual complexity of the agency without foresaking its impact on clients. This comprehensiveness requires four internally related studies: (1) a program goals study; (2) a program implementation study; (3) a program impact study; and (4) an inter-organizational relations or context study. After the program goals have been tentatively determined, the implementation and inter-organizational studies should be conducted with the underlying aim of determining their relation to the impact of the program on the target population. This section will discuss these aspects of advocacy/empowerment program evaluation.

Program goals study

The purpose of the program goals study is to accurately ascertain and formulate the program goals such that the extent to which they are accomplished can be measured. A program whose goals are stated very vaguely and generally, or not at all, cannot be evaluated. Goals must be operationalized in terms that are empirically verifiable to be effective as evaluative criteria.

The purpose of calling this first stage of program evaluation research a goals 'study' is that the program goals are not as easily determined as might first appear. The goals do not necessarily 'exist' somewhere to be discovered, but require a combination of discovery and creation through aggressive research on the part of the evaluator. Of course, the most desirable method of goal formulation is to be involved as a participant in the initial planning phases of the program. If, however, the evaluator comes to the scene later on, he or she should be aware that the ascertainment of the program goals involves much more than merely a listing of them from the program proposal.

In the pursuit of goals as evaluative criteria, it is important to be aware that many organizations have diverse sets of goals, with some participant groups and constituencies having conflicting interests. Thus the choice of a set of goals as the evaluative criteria takes on a normative and political character. In these cases the normative and political bases of goal selection, e.g., whose interests are benefited, should be made explicit by the evaluator (Scott, 1981, p. 324). However, advocacy/empowerment agencies, by definition, are characterized by basic goal consensus. The work of the evaluator then becomes that of discovering how the goals are operationalized.

A useful distinction to be made at the outset of the goals study is between the 'official' and 'operational' goals of a program (Perrow, 1961, p. 855). Official goals are 'the general purposes of the organization as put forth in the charter, annual reports, public statements by key executives, and other authoritative pronouncements.' Operative goals, on the other hand, 'designate the ends sought through the actual operating policies of the organization; they tell us what the organization actually is trying to do, regardless of what the official goals say are the aims' (Perrow, 1961, p. 855). The evaluator should begin by locating the official goals. These might be found in the initial program proposal, mandating legislation, or other formal documents. By successive approximations, the evaluator can then move toward the formulation of the operational goals. Study of the theoretical literature that informs the practice paradigm, repeated interviews with program staff and participant observation are helpful in the formulation of the

Table 7.1 Community Support Systems Program goals

	Program Implementation Goals	Program Impact Goals	Program Inter-organizational Goals
ULTIMATE GOALS	a Integration of theory and practice b Delivery of Adv/ Emp* Service to client population c Validation and support of staff	a Enhance quality of life of clients b Increased autonomy, power, self-respect, community integration, health and welfare of clients	a Client survival and development b Program survival
INTERMEDIATE GOALS	a Establish practice in homes b Establish staff training in Adv/ Emp model c Establish staff group decision process d Gain access to adult homes	a Increased knowledge of legal rights and entitlements b Increased use of community resources c Increased ability to negotiate everyday life in the community d Increased sense of self-worth and citizenship	a Increase quantity and quality of services from agencies in the inter-organizational field b Gain access to adult homes and hotels so as to provide services c Maintain strong relationship with community constituencies d Maintain autonomy from medical model domination
IMMEDIATE GOALS	a Build client population b Begin weekly training sessions c Begin open discussion staff meetings	a Possession of Medicaid card b Knowledge of rights related to housing c Knowledge of right to refuse mental health medication d Knowledge of right to vote	a Advocate for more and better services from supporting agencies at every opportunity b Instigate investigation of access issue c Refuse to become subordinate member of service provider-home owner treatment team

* Advocacy/Empowerment

operational goals. Once these goals are formulated, there should be general agreement amongst program staff as to their accuracy.

A further important goal clarification is the distinction between ultimate, intermediate and immediate goals. In moving from ultimate to immediate goals, there is an increase in the tentativeness and flexibility of the goal. Some of our Community Support Systems Program goals are outlined in Table 7.1.

Program implementation study

Once goals are formulated, research designs for the implementation, impact and inter-organizational studies can be constructed. The implementation research design for our Community Support Systems Program focuses on several issues: (1) Is the paradigm of the program (e.g., problem definition, program goals, and appropriate practice principles and action orientation) being effectively communicated to staff through training?; (2) Do the quality and quantity of the services being delivered embody the program paradigm?; (3) Does the program's group decision making process facilitate communication, validation and involvement with work on the part of staff?; (4) What are the major obstacles to effective implementation?

Four methods of data collection were used to address questions of internal consistency and practice: (1) extensive participant observation during the initial year of the program in the staff in-service training sessions, in the field where services are delivered, and in weekly staff meetings; (2) content analysis of 'client contact sheets' which are summaries of the nature of each client contact filled out each time a case manager has a contact with a client; (3) quantitative analysis of output measures, e.g., monthly 'units of service,' number of clients, etc.; and (4) ongoing open-ended interviews with program staff. The variety of data provides a rich resource from which to evaluate the extent to which the program is being implemented as planned.

Program impact study

The research design for the program impact study requires a causal impact model as well as a data collection design. An impact model is a clear causal statement indicating which variables are going to have what effect on which other variables. Typically, for program evaluation, the impact model states the expected or hypothesized effect or impact of the program (independent) variable – e.g., treatment, training, education, social service, etc. – on the target (dependent) variable – e.g., attitudes or actions of target population. A typical program impact model has the following format:

PROGRAM→→ATTITUDES→→BEHAVIOUR→→CONDITIONS

The impact model for our Community Support Systems Program is shown in Figure 7.1.

Figure 7.1 Community Support Systems Program impact model

Advocacy/Empowerment CSS Services	Increased knowledge of rights and entitlements	Increased acquisition of legal rights
	Increased use of community resources	Increased community integration
	Increased ability to negotiate everyday life in the community	Enhanced quality of life
	Increased sense of self-worth and citizenship	Decreased exploitation and manipulation

Program evaluation research designs to measure program impact range in rigor from the classic experiment, with before and after program measures of control and experimental groups, to 'quasi-experiments' utilizing 'constructed,' non-random, non-equivalent control groups (Campbell, 1969); to 'approximate methods' which do not control for contaminating influences or extraneous confounding factors at all (Rossi *et al.*, 1979, p. 227). Which design is chosen is dependent upon the researcher's purposes, time, resources and available possibilities for the utilization of control groups. It is often morally, politically and logistically impossible to withhold services from a group for research purposes. However, some programs can only serve a small proportion of the eligible population, so that control groups become morally and logistically possible.

For our Community Support Systems Program, randomized control groups are not available since the program serves everyone in the geographic area who is eligible for services and wishes to receive them. The impact design we have chosen is a 'cross sectional' study using statistical controls. Rossi defines a cross sectional study as:

One in which observations are made at a single point in time, contrasting those who have participated in an intervention with those who have not (or who have participated in varying degrees). Usually the population is sampled, and a survey administered to gather information on a large number of possibly confounding variables. Differences between levels of exposure to an intervention are held constant through statistical analysis, along with the other relevant differences between participants and non-participants. (Rossi *et al.*, 1979, p. 214)

We constructed a questionnaire called the 'social profile' (see Appendix VII), and administered it to approximately half of the participants in the program (N = 60), after the program had been in operation for twenty months. In the analysis of the data, comparisons will be made of those groups of participants with differing degrees of exposure to the program by statistically controlling for degree of participation in the program. Program impact questions will be asked, such as: Do those who have a greater degree of program exposure also score higher on knowledge of rights and entitlements, or community integration than do those who have a lesser degree of program exposure?; Does sex, age, race, type of home, hospitalization background or type of medication have an effect on program impact?

A common problem with this design is its inability to take into account the effects of self-selection on the impact of the program. Since all of the interviews are with program participants, possibly there is something about those who decided to be a program participant that significantly differentiates them from those who decided not to become participants. If this were the case, the research design would be unable to take this difference into account in its estimates of program impact. This is not a problem, however, for this study, since 98 per cent of those eligible to receive services in the area have consented to become program participants and are receiving services.

Issues of validity and reliability are particularly relevant for a study involving former mental patients because of their peculiar history. Questions of reliability address whether or not different interviewers or researchers can obtain similar results utilizing the same research instruments, and questions of validity address whether or not any, or all, of the researchers obtain accurate results, results that have some truth value. There is often a tension between reliability and validity as Hyman *et al.* make clear:

In developing a model interviewing procedure, one must somehow balance the gains in reduction of inter-interviewer variability that come from standardization against the possible loss of validity due to the inflexibility of the procedures for the range of circumstances, the constraints placed upon the interviewer's insight, and the loss of informality. One can array various approaches to the literature along the continuum of the freedom allowed the interviewer. Depending on the position of this continuum, one notes that the validity component has presumably been maximized through the exercise of great freedom in interviewing, or that the reliability component has been maximized through standardization of procedure. (Hyman *et al.*, 1954, p. 30)

Whether or not the interview process is standardized or flexible, and whether or not the interviewer attempts to gain 'rapport' with the respondent or remains distant and business-like, misses the more important and basic question of the nature of the *relationship* between interviewer and respondent. How does the respondent view the interviewer? The importance of the relationship aspect of the inter-view process, and its relation to validity, becomes even clearer when the respondents are deinstitutionalized former mental patients. After having spent years in state mental institutions, and having been interviewed countless times by psychiatrists, psychologists, social workers, nurses and others, institutionalized mental patients develop strategies for answering interview questions so as to minimize harm to themselves. In the hospital when they have answered truthfully, e.g., when they have exposed true feelings of anger, confusion or mistrust to interviewers, it was often interpreted as part of their 'illness' and used against them (Goffman, 1961). In response to this, patients' answers increasingly take the form of perfunctory superficiality, passive con-formity and compliance. Thus, when asked questions about horrible living conditions a typical response might be, 'Everything is fine' (Allen, 1974, p. 11).

For a researcher to move beyond this superficial level to a deeper level of response, and thus more valid findings, requires a relationship based upon some sense of trust. The respondent has to know, first, that the information and feelings that he or she shares are not going to be used against him or her in any way in the future, and second, that his or her accounts of the world are seen as valid accounts and not symptoma-tology of illness. This requires a relationship of human being to human being with which, typically, former psychiatric patients have had little recent experience. Without this trusting relationship, however, the information garnered from an interview would be very problematic in terms of validity.

Program evaluation research of our Community Support Systems Program has in large part been able to overcome this obstacle to validity. The CSS program emphasis upon advocacy/empowerment, confidentiality and validation of the person has already nurtured supportive and trustful relationships with many of the participants, and thus, as part of the same program, the researchers were also trusted. In addition, the program researchers spent time in the field doing participant observation. By the time we were ready to begin engaging with participants in the questionnaire-interview process, we either already knew many, if not most, of the program participants, or were, at minimum, strongly associated with the Community Support Systems Program and thus trusted. Where possible, a researcher was paired with a case manager or day program staff member to conduct the interview jointly. As a result of the involvement of the program staff, the research interview took on the functions of further elaborating the client's perspective on the many issues contained in the Social Profile instrument; of identifying individual and aggregate problems and concerns, thus focusing client-centered attention on agenda building for future program activity; and of quality control, since staff could inquire about a client's answers to questions that dealt with material which they had previously discussed.

It is our relationship to the participants of the program that is the single most important factor in ensuring the validity of our questionnaire/interview data. Most program participants, after agreeing to be interviewed, did not hesitate to discuss aspects of their life conditions in an open way. The reliability of our study, or the extent to which our findings could be replicated by other researchers would have to depend not only upon utilization of the same research instrument, the social profile, *but also upon the replication of our research relationship.*

The social profile The social profile has three functions: (1) to aid research; (2) to create potential problem articulation agendas for Community Support Systems staff; and (3) to educate program participants. This section will only address the research functions and the construction and implementation of the social profile. The following section will elaborate on the other two functions.

There are three research purposes of the social profile: (1) to document the conditions of life of the program participants in various areas, e.g., in the adult homes and single room occupancy hotels, medical care, mental health care, finances, transportation, community integration, etc.; (2) to document the extent of the partipants' knowledge of their rights and entitlements; and (3) to document the extent to which the participants are actually receiving their full range of rights and entitlements. The construction of the social profile required two major sets of activities: (1) the ascertainment and compilation of the legal rights and entitlements of *former* mental patients (see Chapter 6); and (2) participant observation fieldwork in the adult homes and single room occupancy hotels with the Community Support Systems staff and program participants in order to gain contextual and concrete understanding of the participants' everyday life round of events, language and perceptions of what is and is not relevant. Once the legal information was compiled, it had to be translated into questions utilizing language that the participants could understand, and phrased in ways that would have relevance to their everyday lives. This translation was a group process that drew upon the experience of everyone in the project.

The implementation process began with our introducing the social profile to the participants, explaining what it was and what its purposes were. Emphasis was placed upon the fact that participation in the interview was strictly a matter of choice on their part, and that all information from the interview would be strictly confidential. Appointments were made and, again, at the time of the individual interview, choice and confidentiality were reiterated. Two people were present at each interview, one to write down the answers verbatim, to free the other to maintain rapport with the interviewee. The non-coercive nature of the interviews and our assurances created a relaxed situation and greatly enhanced the interview experience for all involved, and recreated the relational factor in enhancing validity.

Functions of the social profile for participants and staff   The social profile was designed not just to take information from the program participants, but also to give it. In formulating legal rights and entitlements in question form, the social profile alerts and informs the program participants as to what their rights and entitlements are. The social profile also helps participants to recognize that if these stipulated rights and entitlements are not being received, this is a problem which needs to be solved (Freire, 1970). This educational and problem posing function of the social profile makes it somewhat unwieldy as a research instrument, but contributes greatly towards the atmosphere of the interview as a sharing process.

During the course of the social profile interview many problems are typically identified as relevant to the participant. The identification of these problems serves the purpose of aiding the Community Support Systems staff in constructing agendas within which to pursue follow-up case management work with the participants and since a member of the staff is a co-interviewer with a researcher, the response was immediate.

In these ways, the Community Support Systems Program evaluation has immediate relevance and provides immediate feedback to program participants and staff, rather than existing as just an extra burden of work for them. It is an extension of the ongoing dialogue (Freire, 1970) between staff and clients rather than a process of extraction of information extraneous to both.

Program inter-organizational study

The nature of program contacts with other organizations in the inter-organizational field can have significant effects upon the program's implementation and impact. Our Community Support Systems Program evaluation utilizes several data sources and methods to monitor and document the program's contact with other organizations in the field. They are the following: (1) content analysis of 'Inter-organizational Contact Sheets.' Inter-organizational Contact Sheets are descriptions of the nature and outcome of every contact with another organization by program staff. Our content analysis focuses upon the content of the specific issue; the nature of the issue, e.g., turf, service, and/or ideological; the nature of the contact, e.g., cooperation, contest, or conflict (Warren *et al.*, 1974); and the outcome; (2) content analysis of the inter-organizational correspondence; and (3) participant observation at inter-organizational meetings.

These data and analyses enable us to formulate the nature of the inter-organizational context within which the program operates. Knowledge as to which organizations are willing or unwilling, able or unable, to provide support, and around which issues, is very valuable input into program and/or policy planning. Systematic information on outcomes of the various contacts around the various problems is helpful in the development of advocacy procedures, and thus in the provision of better services to program participants.

This chapter has examined the purposes, pitfalls and procedures of advocacy/empowerment program evaluation. The purposes of enhancing the agency's ability to reflect critically upon itself, to defend itself against inter-organizational attack, and to launch assertive advocacy strategies makes evaluation a central component of the advocacy/empowerment agency, and well worth the investment in resources. Failure to avoid the output, outcome and acontextual pitfalls, however, can lead to erroneous conclusions and an inadvertant reproduction of the dominant ideology or inter-organizational thought structure. This failure can prove very harmful to those agencies that seek to pursue the interests of their clients which are often in conflict with the dominant inter-organizational thought structure. To avoid working in directions counter to the interests of its clients, advocacy/empowerment agencies must use a multidimensional evaluation approach which includes studies of the program goals, implementation process, impact on clients and inter-organizational context. The program evaluation approach of our CSSP is presented as an example of this multidimensional approach, and provides a case study of how some of the more important issues within each of these dimensions might be addressed.

CHAPTER 8

Community Organization

Community-based programs providing services to any client group, and especially to those with social stigma, are placed in an ironic situation: while they are often needed, they are also perceived to be threatening to their host communities. Because many service providing agencies with community-based programs have their funding determined by extra-community sources (state bureaucracies, for example), and because the agencies have rarely been invited into communities, or where invited in, rarely asked to locate where they have by the immediate neighbors, community members, who do not utilize the services offered, frequently feel antagonism toward the agency. When there is a high degree of stigma attached to the clients served, the antagonism frequently rises because community members feel that the agency has brought undesirable characters into town or into the neighborhood. Whether the community's anger is directed towards the clients, the funding agency or the operating agency, the anger felt (but rarely openly expressed) reflects feelings of being out of control of one's immediate environment. Concerns about property values skyrocket as if price and market were determined locally. The operating agency and its clients are held accountable for falling housing markets and perceived, but not recorded, drops in real estate prices.

These faulty beliefs, while not true, nonetheless demonstrate clearly the intensity of the feelings involved. One need only look at the number of homes purchased as non-profit community residences which have been burned down to see a concrete demonstration of the intensity of these feelings. Other tactics indicating the intensity of

community opposition include neighbors banding together to purchase houses being considered for conversion into community residences
for ex-patients. In New York challenges to site location were so
commonplace that legislation was passed requiring public hearings on
site selection and specifying the terms of state control. We believe that
the basis for these feelings is the continuous usurpation of individual
control over crucial issues (e.g., the impact of inflation, unemployment, defense spending, foreign policy, etc.) which ultimately affects
the daily life of all individuals and communities. These feelings of
powerlessness are displaced onto easily identifiable targets and onto
people over whom the 'normal' members of a community feel some
power and status.

Whether an agency is invited (in our case) or uninvited into a
community, the agency is an 'outsider' under any circumstances short
of total community control. 'Outsiders' have played an historic role in
our society, causing suspicions and producing cohesiveness among
'insiders' since the days of the independent colonies. The fear of being
harmed by strangers, especially when those newcomers have the
frightening label of 'mental patient,' reinforces the firmly held tradition of exclusion and containment which surrounds private property.
When these fears are fed by state bureaucratic action, as was clearly
the case in deinstitutionalization with the dumping of ex-patients into
neighborhoods and communities unprepared to accommodate or provide for them, often the ex-patients became the focal point for a good
deal of misdirected agitation and local grievances. However, for
agencies to ignore community hostility and/or fear, or to feel contempt
for 'uneducated' or 'insensitive' community people, is as misdirected
as the contempt of community members towards the ex-patients
dumped in their midst.

Perceiving the social environment as a central variable for practice
naturally falls beyond the purview of medicalized mental health
after-care programs. Communities as social, economic and cultural
entities cannot be understood from within the psychiatric world view
(Panzetta, 1971). Numerous agencies, focused on the medicalized
defects of their clients and the concomitant desire to provide services
to them, have often completely neglected the people and organizations
which comprise the social reality of the everyday environment in which
their clients live. When looking at the deinstitutionalization of
psychiatric patients, this decision or position is even more absurd than
with other community-based programs. Former patients, during the

years of extensive dumping, most often were dropped off in profit-operated, state-licensed facilities of one type or another, or in single room occupancy hotels (SROs) in communities unfamiliar to the ex-patients. It was the exception rather than the rule to find any local services either available or appropriate to the ex-patients' needs. Communities, in turn, had no power or capacity to oppose the dumping. Insidious intrusion by private profit entrepreneurs in the early days of deinstitutionalization has been replaced in more recent years by the state's legal right (in New York State) to establish community residences in neighborhoods vigorously opposed to their presence. Powerless to fight the profiteers or the state and fiscally unable to supply needs services, communities turned against the former patients in their midst. They also developed antagonism toward the state and a deeply felt mistrust of mental health agencies that were perceived to represent the interests of the state, namely, the dumping of more former patients or the rationalizing of discharge policies.

Communities acted in hostile ways with little understanding of the role of the private housing entrepreneur in creating 'saturated,' underserved, pocket ghettoes of socially stigmatized people. Dumping, engendered by economic policies of the state (see Introduction), combined with profiteering in the private housing market (in the form of SROs and adult homes) to produce 'saturated' or 'impacted' communities. The typical circumstances creating community antagonism could not have evolved without the active, though unintended collaboration of both parties.

Without an adequate comprehension of the meaning of 'outsider,' particularly as it relates to suburban and/or rural areas, and without an adequate understanding of the meaning of the social context or community environment to people's lives, mental health after-care programs unintentionally function to enhance local opposition to their clients' presence in communities. Our a priori perception of this contradictory phenomenon of mental health agencies being in communities while ignoring them as socio-cultural settings of great import, coupled with our belief in the necessity for building positive community alliances, led to the creation of a community organization/ development strategy as soon as our program began. Our knowledge about the likelihood of attack from other service providers (Rose, 1972; Warren *et al.*, 1974) related to turf issues combined with what we understood to be vast, unresolvable ideological differences in operating practice paradigms, indicated to us the necessity of building constituency support for our program among individuals and organizations outside the local inter-organizational network of service providers. Quite obviously, given prevailing community antagonism towards a number of these agencies, community organization became a strategic necessity as well as a preferred choice for organizational survival.

Constituency building always begins with an assessment of individuals, organizations, associations and groups in the community who have expressed concern about issues related to the stigmatized population or who may be likely to do so in the future. It is important to contact elected political officials, church or synagogue and civic groups, professional groups and others to introduce the new program or, in the case of existing programs, to keep community members apprised of the direction and efforts of the program. It is equally important to prepare written materials describing the nature of the program, its administrative auspices, its source of funds and its staff. Addresses and telephone numbers should be included with information indicating who to call with regard to certain issues or concerns. When doing constituency building related to socially stigmatized populations, one should anticipate hostility for all of the reasons described above. Rather than counter hostility with condescension, each community person expressing antagonism towards the population in question or the larger social service system (in our case, ex-patients and the mental health system) must be encouraged to elaborate on these feelings and their causes. Community members expressing feelings of being dominated and out of control of what is happening in their community must be supported and their hostility redirected to the proper targets. This effort at redirection is an educational process, requiring data gathering and assembling information about community members' feelings and perceptions about the situation. The data gathering and exploration of feelings approach described above in Chapters 4 and 5 finds further utilization in community work. Elaboration of individuals' feelings and perceptions, thematization, patterning of themes and representations lead to reformulations of problems and potential action strategies.

We have found that eliciting information from people and supporting their feelings of anger (but not the target), creates a positive climate for political education, education geared towards identifying the proper causes of the problems which confront them.

Individuals representing groups or organizations are told that staff from our agency will gladly come to a meeting of their executive board or planning committee and to general membership meetings to discuss our program orientation and, at a thematic level, to support the group's feelings of anger about having so little control over what happens in their community.

The focus of an initial community meeting, whether it is comprised of heads of organizations or the general membership, is the same: a discussion of who created the problems which exist for the community and a discussion of who has benefited from these policies. In our case, we present an overview of the life circumstances of ex-patients living in adult homes and SROs in the community, perhaps attached to some slides showing the facilities (photographic/and/or slide presentations prepared by staff and clients can be effective in demystifying a program, see Chapter 5). A chart similar to the one used on p. 81) is shown to illustrate the complex situation ex-patients face. The problems which arise in the course of daily life for ex-patients are then woven into an explanation of how the agency is attempting to respond. Services delivered are described along with demystification of the funding process.

Based upon these initial meetings with community groups, we search for ways to keep community members involved with our program. We might form an advisory committee of community people or schedule additional informational meetings. Additionally, community members are invited to come to our programs and to interact with staff and participants. This invitation is offered in order to decrease the distance between community members and the former psychiatric patients living in the community and to cut into the stereotype of 'mental patients' created by obsolete mental health practices. Such an invitation also helps cut into the ominous and threatening stereotype that ex-patients have of community members. Each time a meeting is held in the community, the objective is to redirect anger rather than to demean or diffuse it, and to clarify the roles played by various agencies and bureaucracies in determining what occurs in that community.

One-time educational programs for community associations or church groups have more impact subjectively than objectively, though obviously the two are related. The subjective dimension of educational programs relates to the realm of trust and relationship-building which occurs. Most likely, other service providers have not been responsive to community needs or feelings, and medicalized professionals often treat community scepticism with condemnation. Looking to respond to community anger, stretching to understand its concrete and subjective bases, acting to stimulate dialogue, all produce positive outcomes in relation to building a support system in the locality.

Responsiveness to community concerns can be a way of beginning the process of political education, of transforming feelings of community hostility towards stigmatized populations into a more active, accurate and systemic critique of the particular bureaucratic system and policies which led to the placing of powerless people in communities which were never involved in the planning process. In addition, this process of political education involves looking critically at various individuals and groups within the community who have benefited from such policies. This latter objective is more difficult because it requires a willingness on the part of community people to look critically at individuals or groups who may be benefiting at the expense of the larger community. In the case of our program, this strategy meant looking critically at the mental health system, deinstitutionalization and entrepreneur/landlords benefiting at the expense of former patients. Over time, community members, hopefully, will come to see that the problems faced by former patients are not based simply on the ex-patients' individual frailty or on the inefficiency in the service system, but rather flow from the combination of profit-centered and medicalized definitions of need. Once lay people in the community understand even a small part of this larger contextual reality, their capacity to understand inter-organizational conflict increases as does their ability to understand an advocacy/empowerment approach on the part of an agency such as ours.

An advocacy/empowerment-oriented program, as a strategy to solicit long term support, must learn something about local politics. Program staff must also understand local politics in order to avoid inadvertently getting caught in potentially detrimental political squabbles or provoking long-standing local antagonisms. Bi-partisan and ecumenical organizing, which sticks assiduously to issues that have impact on clients' needs, agency services and the quality of life for former patients, is critical. An important step is to organize a group, committee or association made up of community group members and agency staff. The purpose of such a group is to nurture and develop community support and constituencies. The group must be given a name (ours has been called CASA, for Community After-Care Services Association) for purposes of easy identification and community visibility. It is in the interests of such a group to maintain close contact with locally elected political officials and to know their support groups.

The agency-community group, which might include representatives from other service providers, serving the same target population in the geographic area, becomes the focal point for discussing problems which exist in the community. The group can engage in efforts to problem-solve; it can serve as an information clearing house; it can anticipate forthcoming policy issues and can obtain material for review from distant bureaucracies which impact on agency practice and/or on clients' lives (but which generally go unknown by community people); it can focus attention on and invite representatives from other sub-systems which have impact on clients' lives (e.g., SSI or Medicaid) to attend meetings to explain their agency's role; it can work to bring common community problems to the fore (e.g., the need to develop an emergency plan for housing people in case of fire) and it can expose community people to the conflict situations which regularly confront advocacy/empowerment-oriented agencies.

An agency which creates such a group or association has responsibility for providing leadership to it. Leadership must take several forms, one part of which is simple logistics (for example, making up name, address and telephone lists for everyone, arranging meetings and making sure everyone has transportation). Leadership also expresses itself, especially in early meetings, through implementation of the same principles of group responsibility used in day programs (see Chapter 5): issue clarification through elaboration, thematization, development of thematic patterns and problematization moving on to action strategies and critical assessment. In the form of education, issues related to the lives of clients are introduced, discussions initiated, and preliminary exploration of feelings and thoughts engendered. For major issues, study committees or sub-groups are formed, led by agency staff members. Issues are investigated further and elaborated. Position papers may also be prepared which can be brought to the larger group for deliberation and action.

Drawing from our own experience, our agency-community group (known as CASA) developed a policy paper on After-Care Rights and Responsibilities. This paper began as a discussion at an Agency-Community Association meeting where staff introduced some of the daily life problems and issues confronted by former patients. The issues were referred to a sub-group headed by agency staff for development and elaboration. Eventually, the sub-group returned to the whole Association with a draft of a position paper for representation, refinement and approval. The discussions provoked by the draft document led to significantly broadened perceptions among community people about such issues as homeowner domination, medication, regulating agencies, etc. Drawing on the work of the sub-group, the entire Association then approved the final position paper, drafts of which were prepared by agency staff, as summaries of sub-group discussions. Action strategies were then offered which, in this case, led eventually to a set of legislative hearings and recommendations. Community people were thus able to begin to understand political action as a process of critical analysis and were able to see systemic characteristics which previously were hidden.

The reaction of other service providers to Agency-Community Association group position papers further develops the community participants' consciousness of the inter-organizational context within which services are delivered. This process of expanding awareness of inter-organizational issues is furthered through regularly inviting selected community representatives to all interagency meetings, with particular emphasis on their attendance when conflict-laden issues are most likely to emerge. It is crucial for community representatives to participate in these meetings because the actual experience of inter-agency confrontation, the opportunity to hear other service providers articulate their positions, and the presence of community people itself all contribute to community constituency building. Briefing of community people before such meetings, while helpful, is not nearly so important as 'de-briefing' afterwards. Hearing their accounts afterwards and correcting any distortions is important in order to ensure that the meeting makes as much sense as possible. The likelihood of community people fully understanding the bases for conflict is not great without this type of agency leadership. Over time, through discussions of what took place and why certain things happened at such meetings, community people can begin to see reality from the perspective of the advocacy–empowerment program.

The process of carefully explaining inter-organizational clashes to community participants invited to interagency meetings is crucial in the early stages of community development. In our case, for example, community people could not understand why the staff of the local mental health clinic felt so antagonistic toward advocacy/empowerment agency staff over the issue of confidentiality. Hospital and clinic staff were continually exchanging information about clients with one another, as well as with adult homeowners or SRO management. We absolutely refused to participate in this medium of exchange. The situation became so heated at the local level that we chose to escalate the issue out of the local inter-organizational arena to the Regional Office of the State Office of Mental Health. All participating agencies were told to come to a meeting at the Regional Office. We participated, but only on the condition that at least one community representative from our CASA organization could attend. The mental health providers took the expected position of expediency, arguing for sharing of client information among mental health professionals. The presumption was that ethical conduct in this situation exists simply because professionals are involved. We refused to cooperate, to the point of making it clear that even unanimous agreement of the whole group would have no bearing on our position. The relative insignificance of mental health policy when compared to constitutional law was made as the basis for our view. The community representatives, after the meeting, had to be informed of the assumptions behind each position, and each agency's role in the conflict had to be elaborated in significant detail for the community people to comprehend the basis of the conflict and its meaning. This type of time-consuming activity is required if knowledge and trust are to be built. Simple, rhetorical repudiation of the other agencies is transparent self-aggrandizement and will produce estrangement among community people just as quickly as other forms of transparent self-righteousness.

Careful cultivation of the community support, in the context of a hostile inter-organizational environment, can also prove to be effective in advocacy efforts. Joining in preparation of position papers can lead to authoring legislative testimony jointly, co-presenting at legislative or administrative hearings, making written comments on state, city or county agency policies, regulations and/or guidelines. Forwarding copies of positions on issues to all locally elected representatives can produce impact, or have that potential. Efforts to establish contact with local representatives at city, county or state legislative offices is directly connected to the community organization and legislative advocacy efforts. When elected officials see position papers and written commentaries from an Association in their district, and they know that the community people serving as members of the organization hold offices in other, larger community groups (e.g., civic or neighborhood associations, church social action committees, etc.), the potential impact can be significant. Locally elected representatives often hold no positive view of mental health system track records, and can often be looked to for consultation on and/or sponsorship of legislation. They also can be seen as potential allies in conflict situations with state hospitals and/or other service providers. Keeping these officials updated on local activities of importance retains their interest and sustains their support. It can also present them with useful positions on issues of community importance that, in turn, can add to their own local support.

Marked progress in community organization is shown by growing consciousness among community people of the difference between the advocacy/empowerment program and other service providers in definition of clients' needs or problem definitions, practice principles, appreciation of community context, and by their increased concern about ex-patients' well-being in the community. Community members can be invited into adult homes or any other facility by residents, and facilitating such visits promotes an increased capacity among community people to understand former patients' daily life. In crisis situations, when landlords and homeowners deny access to workers, community people who have developed relationships with residents can become involved as active and especially effective participants in the struggle against landlord domination. Maintaining contact with residents in the homes can be vital sources of support both for them and for workers. The possibility of community involvement in a struggle, which may later become an issue for legislation (see Chapter 6), contributes to the further isolation of landlords from sources of community support. It also forces community people to observe the role played by other agencies: which agencies stand firm behind residents' rights, which side with landlords?

In instances where legal protections are non-existent or vague, such as was the case with landlord domination of SRO residents in New York, community people can play an active political advocacy role representing both residents and the agency vis-à-vis landlords. Taking an active role in demanding code compliance, in insisting on adequate health and safety measures, or food preparation, community people can use political influence where legal avenues, agency input or resident organizing efforts break down. Threatening to investigate tax assessments on SRO buildings, using local political contacts to explore zoning ordinance compliance for every piece of the landlord's property, or even organizing demonstrations to close an SRO and relocate residents properly all put pressures on landlords which promote clients' interests, especially in situations where residents can be directly involved in the action with community members.

In our area, a local SRO landlord, for example, refused to make even minimum alterations in his hotel to produce legally specified levels of heat and hot water. Complaints by residents and by program staff to county health and safety inspectors produced little positive impact – at best, a very short term response. A number of community people, including several civic association members whose homes were near the SRO, were then brought together to meet with SRO residents at the day program. After hearing the residents' story, supported by workers' accounts of their own observations inside the SRO and their efforts to produce code compliance (all carefully documented as to time, nature of complaint, agency and staff person called), the community group, with the SRO residents' permission, decided to talk with the landlord about the complaints. The outcome of the meeting was a schedule for remedying each problem with these rectifications monitored by a community member. Other actions followed: one of the community people who visited the SRO, a member of our Program-Community Association, insisted that the Association invite representatives from the County Health Department to its next meeting to explain the role of the Health Department in regulating SROs. The Health Department explained their legal responsibility for code compliance, they identified pertinent law, and a mechanism for cooperative action was agreed to by Association members and the visiting officials. The community people, then returned to the day program, related the outcome of their meeting with Health Department officials to residents of the SRO and to other participants, thus demonstrating that an active, positive interaction could be achieved between former patients, community members and local governmental officials.

Critical appraisal of a process such as this is a step which must be taken and initiated by program leadership. The purpose of recounting the steps in the process is political education: the conditions in the home are reflected upon and connected to the way the residents are forced to live; income levels are reviewed, and the amount of SSI dollars going to the landlord are compared to the spending allowances available to people; the items which each resident must purchase from the meager leftovers (after rent) are reviewed; the impact of living this way on self-image and self-confidence is posed as a question to the people. Through this process, community people, whose initial political posture is often one of moral outrage, can be engaged in advocacy/empowerment and led to reflect on the oppressive conditions producing the advocacy issue. Through the process of critical reflection, the significance of community advocacy activity takes on deeper meaning to those involved. Community people become better able to see the advocacy/empowerment agency and its approach to practice more clearly, that is, the agency's intentions, its approach to problem definition and its ways of relating to clients. As this process unfolds, the perspective on other agencies in the inter-organizational system also sharpens, thus strengthening the agency-community alliance.

Once a program has reason to believe that its principles and practice orientation are at least partially understood and accepted by constituencies in its host community, the role of community groups can be expanded. A positive relationship with a neighborhood or community civic association, which has the largest and most representative membership, can lead to a commitment from the agency to get association approval prior to any major changes or expansion of program activities. Meeting with some regularity with association executive board members, or on an as-needed basis, program directors can provide a continuous funnel of information to association directors, solicit input from them where appropriate, and maintain continuous communication. Where agency decisions related to funding arise, association members can be informed well in advance about the contract process as well as about who has the decision-making power. Any problems in funding requiring a meeting with staff people from a funding source should include community representatives from the Association as well. In funding crises, the relationship between agency staff and community association members, if characterized by honesty and shared experience, can lead to active community support in the form of demands for sustained funds, community advocacy for the agency and political pressure applied to continue funding. Our program has enjoyed all of these benefits, because of our commitment to doing the community development work in the manner described above.

Our experience has been that at first, community people rarely want to know the detail necessary to understand the complexity of creating and operating any community-based program, much less a program constructed out of an alternative (advocacy/empowerment) paradigm. However, agency staff who are genuinely open to dialogue, interested in learning community members' thoughts and feelings about issues, and free from typical professional condescension, can open possibilities for a more sustained and developed agency-community relationship. When staff of an advocacy/empowerment-based agency reflect on their rather tenuous position within the local inter-organizational field and recall that there will be no support forthcoming from that system, transferring energy, resources and commitment to constituency building among organizations, associations and individuals in the host community becomes a preferred activity as well as a necessary strategy for survival.

Communities are the settings or environments where people participate in daily life. Integration of the ex-patients into their social environments as people or citizens, rather than as aberrations, deviants or medicalized objects depends upon an agency being able to develop a context where the existing community anger, stereotypes and distances can be confronted. Equally important in recognizing the social reality of deinstitutionalization and the provision of services to stigmatized populations is the awareness of what it means to be in a 'host' community, and what community people's feelings are about the issues related to an agency, its clients or its imagery. The larger context for conceptualizing these matters is the shrinking role both individuals and localities have in making critical decisions that affect daily life. In addition, community people have to deal with the fears engendered by the 'mentally ill,' fears derived from the use of institutionalization as a treatment of first resort for the many years preceding deinstitutionalization.

We have attempted to demonstrate that the same practice principles and social action approach used in our direct practice can be used also to develop a community organization strategy. The strategy must provide a base for developing a constituency of support within the community if the program is to survive; it must develop an approach to political education which will support taking issues into advocacy arenas for legal, political and/or legislative action; and it must struggle to cultivate an understanding among involved community people of the practice approaches and problem definitions held by the agency. This latter dimension is produced as part of an ongoing effort to help community people break down the barriers between them and the ex-patients residing in their community. This struggle, in turn, emerges as community people are able to transform stereotypes and widely-held medicalized perceptions into concrete understandings of ex-patients as socially human, subjugated and powerless. Thus the community organization approach advocated here is one which does not simply see community people and/or organizations as useful objects to be manipulated for agency objectives, but rather sees direct corollaries between the community and the ex-patients: both are dominated by external forces, often not directly known (e.g., why does inflation rise faster than income? How does X community benefit from defense spending?); both have decreased power to determine what happens in their immediate environments (e.g., the use of eminent domain to locate a community residence for developmentally disabled adults around the corner, despite the unanimous opposition of neighbors); and both are subject to manipulation by government and media.

Seeing parallels at a thematic level between community members and ex-patients allows for the creation of an organizing strategy which is devoid of objectification and contempt, which encourages community people to express their feelings and doubts, which mandates agency leadership in the representation and connection of this antagonism to the larger social reality. Such a strategy totally contradicts community members' past experiences with state mental health authorities, service providers and entrepreneurial landlords by encouraging community input into issues relevant to their concerns; by attempting to figure out quick responses to problems experienced by community residents relating to the ex-patient population; by bringing people together in an organization to learn about information and policies generally kept hidden from them; by requiring community involvement in interagency settings where previously negotiated arrangements were worked out and mystified by professionals; and by asking community members to know something about the reality experienced by the ex-patients living in their community so that together they can act to change this reality. The community organizing strategy also parallels the direct service strategy in its reformulation of problems, identification of potential action strategies, and critical assessments of actions undertaken. As community people experience the principles involved in a practice where they, too, are the participants, their capacity to comprehend and consciously support the program's work with ex-patients is enhanced.

Community organization thus develops as both a desired and necessary activity. It has aspects related to program development, to organizational survival and to social change. Community organization exists as a form of practice which analyzes the needs of the target population for an adequate social life and struggles to produce the contextual and relational climate in which ex-patients can feel themselves welcomed as persons in their communities.

Conclusion

Our purpose has been to develop an advocacy/empowerment theory of practice and to demonstrate its viability as an approach to practice in several different practice areas. We have seen this orientation work. We have seen both staff and clients benefit from its commitments to human social development and social change. We believe that the advocacy/empowerment approach can replace the vestigial models of 'treatment' which remain and reproduce themselves everywhere. And, ironically, we believe that the practice design we have discussed above can simultaneously be more effective and efficient.

As we have described, an innovative program requires far more than a belief in a new type of theory and practice to sustain itself. The array of conventional agencies whose domains and ideologies are threatened by an innovative program will attempt to contain, coopt or kill off new programs or organizations with advocacy/empowerment orientations. The newcomer to the inter-organizational field will succumb, we believe, unless the program begins its work with a clear-cut formulation of inter-organizational conflict.

Since the lynchpin of almost every community-based mental health program proclaiming the need for comprehensive service delivery for former patients is inter-organizational cooperation, collaboration and coordination, our advice – to pay heed to conflict as an organizing principle – may seem peculiar. But, reading this book, we hope some clarity about this urgent message has emerged. Agencies and workers promoting a medicalized model of mental health treatment as the basis for community-based services function to reproduce both themselves and mental patient identity subjectively while enhancing the positions of dominators and exploiters objectively. The very existence of a 'treatment team' with psychiatrically-oriented mental health workers, social service workers and proprietary home owners lends credence to our contention. Workers socialized into the power and false charity of medicalized models of care are similarly socialized into dominated power relationships with clients which are dependent upon the client remaining within the crushing, stultifying confines of the mental patient role. When an advocacy/empowerment practice asserts the oppression in that role, the fight for competing legitimacies erupts at every level, beginning with direct face-to-face contact with clients exposed to both orientations and continuing on to homeowners, regulatory agencies and funding systems. The very life of the advocacy/empowerment agency is regularly put on the line, so long as it maintains its espoused commitments.

In the face of the anticipated attacks, both overt and covert, which inevitably come, the advocacy/empowerment agency must stake out the terms of its own survival. This prerequisite for continued, non-coopted operation is dependent upon continuous commitment of resources to community organization and development – as described in the last chapter. It extends to converting some staff time and energy from direct practice into program evaluation, particularly that part of the evaluation focused on inter-organizational relations, and to careful monitoring of the quality of work done by staff in filling out the forms and data-gathering protocols. Survival further requires that administrative staff spend a good deal of time in meetings with community constituencies educating them to the conflict-ridden realities of existence, and involving those constituencies in inter-organizational meetings and confrontations.

What we have argued is that resolution of conflicts with service provider agencies simply will not occur so long as the advocacy/empowerment agency maintains its beliefs and the other agency remains embedded in some form of psychiatric world view. The absence of overt conflict, or even collaborating on an issue with another agency (for example, advocating with the State Office of Mental Health to issue reimbursement cheques to the contracting agencies in a rational, non-debilitating time frame) does not indicate the resolution of inter-organizational conflict. These situations simply suggest a momentary absence of an issue provoking the intense antagonism inherent in the conflict.

In the chapters above, particularly in the material on community constituency building and legislative advocacy, we have suggested that the support base for an advocacy/empowerment program is to be found outside the service delivery system at both the local and extra-community levels. Again, this strategy is based on the belief that agencies exist not only in a concrete social structural location (organization domain or turf), but in an institutionalized thought structure (Warren *et al.*, 1974) as well. Where competition over various aspects of turf is to be expected, equally predictable are the strategies used by the contenders. These strategies will be invoked to fight over resources, but not to the extent that one agency, or a group of agencies, attempts to terminate totally the existence of their adversary. This latter level of conflict is engendered only when the new agency or program is ideologically in contradiction to the other organizations in the inter-organizational field (Warren *et al.*, 1974). The advocacy/empowerment organization, which takes problems out of an individual defect program model, and redefines problems in order to understand people as oppressed human beings living and enduring socially understandable and potentially alterable conditions, produces the type of ideological contradiction we are referring to.

The task of people struggling to build an advocacy/empowerment-oriented program is to recognize that the nature of interagency conflict is enduring; that its essence is irreconcilable differences and that its character is dramatically different from forms of organizational behavior typically taught in colleges and universities. Differences in ideological framework require differences in perception of program purposes and possibilities; differences in perception of clients' identities and potentials; and differences in the composition of support networks. Where conventional agencies will always turn to their horizontal inter-organizational field, or to the vertical system (local-regional-state offices of the same delivery system) of which they are a part, the advocacy/empowerment agency must act differently. It must create its own constituencies from among people, agencies and associations who have no stake in either the social structural position of the conventional agencies, nor in their obsolete paradigms of practice. Where the conventional agencies will use conventional methods to usurp the advocacy/empowerment agency's resources or legitimation, the advocacy/empowerment agency must resort to unconventional practices to survive. Such practices include refusing to participate in inter-organizational meetings without community members present; giving community constituencies access to programs and policies usually not available to them; introducing community members and clients to one another and working to build compatibility between them; challenging the profit sector and its interests and pointing out conflict of interest situations such as the joint agency-homeowner 'treatment team'; challenging the validity of discharge plans which have no valid information about the objective reality faced by the patient upon leaving the hospital; or refusing to agree to share information unless the requesting client has fully informed consent. Seeking legislative and legal supports and strategies of conventional attack furthers the distance between conventional agencies and advocacy/empowerment-oriented programs. Conventional agencies typically confine their world of practice to their own domains and within the hegemony of their turf, therefore, they can see no possible situations requiring an adversarial posture.

Whatever the particulars of a situation may be, the constants transcend them: conflict is a survival strategy. To fail to understand the true nature of inter-organizational relations is to pave the way for the demise of the advocacy/empowerment program, either through succumbing to active attack or through erosion via cooptation. The nature of the reality is harsh, parallel to the lives of the people in whose interests the advocacy/empowerment program has been created. To forget to attend to the conflict inherent in the advocacy/empowerment position because it is unfamiliar, awkward or threatening to advocacy/empowerment staff is to betray the people and to mystify the class privilege which allows the workers to shrug their shoulders in either coopted victory (the legitimation given to advocacy/empowerment agencies that concede) or in defeat. The issue, guiding our work with clients, is the struggle to transform the objective conditions of oppression as they exist, and in the struggle, to create ourselves.

IT-214

NY State
Tax Department

New York State
Claim For Real Property Tax Credit
for Homeowners and Renters

1982

Page 1

R

PRINT OR TYPE				
First name and initial (if joint claim, enter both names)		Last name		Your social security number
Home address (number and street or rural route)			Apt. No.	Spouse's social security number
City, village or post office	State		ZIP code	NY State county of residence
Full address of New York residence that qualifies you for this credit, if different from above. If not, enter "same."				

If you live in a nursing home or public housing project, enter its name **1**

Including yourself, how many members of your household are filing Form IT-214? Enter number. **2a**

Were any of these household members (or your spouse, if this is a joint claim) 65 or older on December 31, 1982? **2b** ☐ Yes ☐ No

Were you a New York State resident for the entire taxable year? **3** ☐ Yes ■ No

Did you occupy the same residence for at least six months during 1982? **4** ☐ Yes ■ No

Can you be claimed as a dependent on another taxpayer's 1982 federal return? **5** ■ Yes ☐ No
(If you checked a shaded box on line 3, 4 or 5, stop; you do not qualify for this credit.)

Did you own or pay rent for your residence during 1982? **6** ☐ Own ☐ Rent

Enter real property taxes paid **or** 25% of adjusted rent paid *(from page 2, line 28, 32 or 34)* **7**

Enter household gross income from page 2, line 24. *(If this amount is more than $16,000, stop; you do not qualify for this credit.)* **8**

Enter from this table the rate that applies to your household gross income. **9**

RATE TABLE	If the amount on line 8 is:	Your rate is:	If the amount on line 8 is:	Your rate is:
	$0 to $3,600	.040	$ 5,401 to $10,000	.055
	$3,601 to $5,400	.045	$10,001 to $16,000	.065

Multiply line 8 by line 9; enter the result. **10**

Subtract line 10 from line 7 *(If line 10 is more than line 7, stop; no credit is allowed.)* **11**

If you checked the **YES** box on line 2b, the **OWN** box on line 6 and the amount on line 8 is $7,200 or less, enter 25% of line 11 **OR** If you do **not** meet all three conditions, enter 50% of line 11. **12**

If you checked the **YES** box on line 2b and the amount on line 8 is $7,200 or less, enter $250 **OR** $7,201 or more, enter $100 **OR** If you checked the **NO** box on line 2b, enter $45. **13**

Enter the amount from line 12 **OR** 13, whichever is **less**. This is the credit for your household. **14**
(If more than one member of your household is filing Form IT-214, see line 14 instructions.)

- If you are filing a New York State income tax return, transfer the amount on line 14 of this form to Form IT-200, line 14 or to Form IT-201, line 20, whichever you are filing. Attach this claim form to your return.
- If you are not filing a return, mail this form to: NY State Income Tax, State Campus, Albany, NY 12227.

Your signature	Spouse's signature (if joint claim)	Date	For office use only
Paid preparer's signature and address		Date	

IT-214 (1982)   **Page 2**

Get **free assistance** at your local New York State district tax office. Bring all necessary information to complete Schedules A and D (including social security numbers), and either Schedule B or Schedule C below.

───────────────── **Schedule A — Household Gross Income** ─────────────────

Enter the amounts, even if not taxable, that you and all members of your household received during 1982.

How many people lived in your household during 1982? Enter number and complete Schedule D.	**15**	
Federal adjusted gross income *(from Form 1040A, line 12, Form 1040EZ, line 3 or Form 1040, line 32)*. If you do not have to file a federal return, enter the amount which would be included in federal adjusted gross income if a federal return had been required.	**16**	
NY State additions to federal adjusted gross income	**17**	
Social security payments	**18**	
Supplemental security income payments (SSI)	**19**	
Pensions and annuities not included on lines 16 through 19	**20**	
Cash public assistance and relief	**21**	
Unemployment compensation not included on line 16	**22**	
Other income	**23**	
Household gross income *(add lines 16 through 23)*. Enter this amount here, then round to the nearest whole dollar and enter on page 1, line 8	**24**	

───────────────── **Schedule B — Real Property Taxes Paid** ─────────────────

Homeowners — *Enter the amounts you and all qualified members of your household paid during 1982.*

Real property taxes *(including school district taxes)*	**25**	
Special assessments	**26**	
Amounts exempted from taxation under Section 467 of the Real Property Tax Law, for persons 65 years or older	**27**	
Real property taxes paid *(add lines 25 through 27)*. Enter here and on page 1, line 7	**28**	

───────────────── **Schedule C — Rent Constituting Real Property Taxes Paid** ─────────────────

*If your residence was 100% exempt from real property taxes, **stop**; you do not qualify for this credit.*

Renters—Complete lines 29 through 32 only if your 1982 rent payments included heat, gas, electricity, furnishings, or board and if none of these charges were separately stated. If your rent payments did not include any of these charges, go directly to line 33.

Enter the rent you and all members of your household paid during 1982.	**29**	
If line 29 includes charges for heat, **or** heat and gas, enter 15% of line 29 **OR** If line 29 includes charges for heat, gas, and electricity, enter 20% of line 29 **OR** If line 29 includes charges for heat, gas, electricity, and furnishings, enter 25% of line 29 **OR** If line 29 includes charges for heat, gas, electricity, furnishings, and board, enter 50% of line 29	**30**	
Adjusted rent *(subtract line 30 from line 29; if over $300 in any one month, **stop**; you do not qualify)*	**31**	
Enter 25% of line 31 here and on page 1, line 7	**32**	
Enter rent you and all members of your household paid during 1982; do **not** include charges for heat, gas, electricity, furnishings, or board *(If over $300 in any one month, **stop**; you do not qualify)*	**33**	
Enter 25% of line 33 here and on page 1, line 7	**34**	

───────────────── **Schedule D — Household Members** ─────────────────

Name	Social security number	Age	Name	Social security number	Age

1982 Instructions For Form IT-214
Claim For Real Property Tax Credit

NY State
Tax Department

Real Property Tax Credit

If your household gross income was $16,000 or less, you may be entitled to a credit on your New York State income tax return for part of the real property taxes or rent you paid during 1982. If you do not have to file a return, you can file for a refund of the credit by using Form IT-214 only.

Who Qualifies

Homeowners – To qualify for the real property tax credit, you have to meet all of these conditions for the taxable year 1982.

☐ Your household gross income was $16,000 or less.

☐ You occupied the same New York residence for six months or more.

☐ You or your spouse paid real property taxes on your residence.

☐ You were a New York State resident for all of 1982.

☐ You could not be claimed as a dependent on someone else's federal income tax return.

☐ Your residence was not completely exempted from real property taxes.

☐ The current market value of all your real property (house, garage, land, etc.) was $65,000 or less.

☐ Any rent you received for nonresidential use of your residence was 20 percent or less of the total rent you received.

Renters – To qualify for the real property tax credit, you have to meet all of these conditions for the taxable year 1982.

☐ Your household gross income was $16,000 or less.

☐ You occupied the same New York residence for six months or more.

☐ You or your spouse paid rent for your residence.

☐ You were a New York State resident for all of 1982.

☐ You could not be claimed as a dependent on someone else's federal income tax return.

☐ Your residence was not completely exempted from real property taxes.

☐ The rent you and other members of your household paid was $300 or less each month, not counting charges for heat, gas, electricity, furnishings or board.

If you meet all of these conditions, you are a qualified taxpayer and may be entitled to the real property tax credit.

Which Form to File

To claim the real property tax credit, complete Form IT-214, *Claim For Real Property Tax Credit*, and attach it to your return. If neither you nor your spouse has to file a New York return but you qualify to claim the credit, just file Form IT-214 to claim your credit payment.

If more than one member of your household qualifies for the credit, each must file a separate Form IT-214. However, if you are married and filing a joint tax return, you must file a joint claim on Form IT-214.

You cannot file a claim for a taxpayer who has died.

When to File

If you are filing a New York State income tax return, attach Form IT-214 to it and file both as soon as you can after January 1, 1983, but not later than April 15, 1983.

If you don't have to file a New York State income tax return, file Form IT-214 as soon as you can after January 1, 1983.

Privacy Act Notification

The Federal Privacy Act of 1974, as amended, requires all agencies requesting identifying numbers to inform individuals from whom they seek information why the request is being made and how the information is used.

The disclosure of identifying numbers, including social security numbers, is required by Section 171-a of the Tax Law and by Section 152.1 of the Personal Income Tax Regulations. Such numbers which are disclosed on any report or return or which your employer lawfully furnishes to this department are used for tax administration purposes and as necessary pursuant to Education Law Section 663, Social Services Law Sections 23, 111-b and 136-a, Executive Law Section 49, Tax Law Sections 171-a, 171-b, 171-c, 171-d and 697 and Labor Law Section 537 and when the taxpayer gives written authorization to this department for another department, person, agency or entity to have access, limited or otherwise, to information contained in his return.

Definitions

All who share your residence, and its furnishings, facilities and accommodations are **members of your household**, whether they are related to you or not.

Household members also include tenants, subtenants, roomers or boarders if they are **related** to you in any of the following ways:

– A son, daughter or a descendent of either.
– A stepson or stepdaughter.
– A brother, sister, stepbrother or stepsister.
– A father, mother or an ancestor of either.
– A stepfather or stepmother.
– A niece or nephew.
– An aunt or uncle.
– A son-in-law, daughter-in-law, father-in-law, mother-in-law, brother-in-law or sister-in-law.

No one can be a member of more than one household at one time.

Household gross income is the total of the following income items that you and all members of your household received:

☐ Federal adjusted gross income (even if you don't have to file a federal return).

☐ New York State additions to federal adjusted gross income. For a list of these additions, see Publication 308, *Real Property Tax Credit*, or page 14 of the instructions for Form IT-201.

☐ Any part of the following items of income **not** included in either of the above.

– Pensions and annuities, including railroad retirement benefits, all payments received under the federal Social Security Act and veterans' disability pensions.
– All state unemployment insurance payments.
– Support money.
– Gain from the sale or exchange of property.
– Disability benefits excluded by Section 105(d) of the Internal Revenue Code.
– Income earned abroad exempted by Section 911 of the Internal Revenue Code.
– Supplemental Security Income (SSI) payments.
– Nontaxable interest received from New York State, its agencies, instrumentalities, public corporations or political subdivisions.
– Workers' compensation.
– The gross amount of **loss-of-time** insurance.
– Cash public assistance and relief, other than medical assistance for the needy.
– Nontaxable strike benefits.

Household gross income does not include surplus food or other relief in kind.

A **residence** is a dwelling that you own or rent, and up to one acre of land around it. It must be located in New York State. If your residence is on more than one acre of land, only the amount of real property taxes or rent paid that applies to the residence and only one acre around it may be used to figure the credit. (If you do not know how much real or real property tax you paid for the one acre surrounding your residence, contact your local assessor.) Each residence within a multiple dwelling unit may qualify. A condominium, a cooperative or a rental unit within a single dwelling is also a residence.

A trailer or mobile home that is used only for residential purposes and is defined as real property under the Real Property Tax Law is also a residence.

Real property taxes paid are all real property taxes, special ad valorem levies and assessments levied and paid upon a residence owned or previously owned by a qualified taxpayer (or spouse, if the spouse occupied the residence for at least six months) during the taxable year. Real property taxes paid include amounts exempted from tax under Section 467 (for persons 65 and older) of the Real Property Tax Law. If you do not know this amount, contact your local assessor.

Real property taxes paid also include any real estate taxes allowed (or which would be allowable if the taxpayer had filed returns on a cash basis) as a deduction for tenant-stockholders in a cooperative housing corporation under Section 216 of the Internal Revenue Code.

If any part of your residence was owned by someone who was not a member of your household, include only those real property taxes paid that apply to the part you and other qualified members of your household own.

If your residence was part of a larger unit, include only the amount of real property taxes paid that can be reasonably applied to your residence.

If you owned and occupied more than one residence during the taxable year, add together the prorated part of real property taxes paid for the period you occupied each residence.

Rent constituting real property taxes paid is 25 percent of the adjusted rent paid on a New York residence during the taxable year after subtracting any charges for heat, gas, electricity, furnishings or board. If these charges are not separately stated, complete lines 29 through 32 of Schedule C of Form IT-214 to figure 25 percent of adjusted rent. Do not include any subsidized part of your rental charge in adjusted rent.

If any part of your residence was rented by someone who was not a member of your household, include on line 29 of Form IT-214 only the amount of rent you and members of your household paid.

If you moved from one rented residence to another rented residence during the taxable year, add 25 percent of adjusted rent paid for each residence.

Line-by-Line Instructions — Form IT-214

Print or type the information requested in the name and address box at the top of page 1. Enter your name, address, social security number and county of residence as of December 31, 1982. Married taxpayers enter both social security numbers. On the bottom line of the name and address box, enter the address of the New York residence that qualifies you for this credit if it is different from your mailing address. If not, enter the word "same" on this line.

Line 1

If you were a resident of a nursing home or a public housing project, enter its name.

Line 2a

Enter the number of members of your household, including yourself, who are filing a Form IT-214 for 1982. Count a joint claim filed by husband and wife as one Form IT-214.

Line 2b

If any qualified member of your household was 65 or older on December 31, 1982, check the **Yes** box. If not, check the **No** box.

Line 3

If you were a New York State resident for all of 1982, check the **Yes** box. If not, check the **No** box.

Line 4

If you occupied the same residence for six months or more during 1982, check the **Yes** box. If not, check the **No** box.

Line 5

If you can be claimed as a dependent on someone else's 1982 federal income tax return, check the **Yes** box. If not, check the **No** box.

If you checked a shaded box on line 3, 4 or 5, **stop**; you do not qualify for this credit.

Line 6

If you owned your residence, check the **Own** box. If you paid rent for your residence, check the **Rent** box. If you owned your residence for part of the year and rented your residence for part of the year, check the **Own** box.

Line 7

Real Property Taxes Paid or 25 Percent of Adjusted Rent Paid

If you owned your residence for all of 1982, complete Schedule B on page 2 of Form IT-214, using the instructions below.

If you rented your residence for all of 1982, complete Schedule C on page 2 of Form IT-214, using the instructions below.

If you owned your residence for part of the taxable year and rented your residence for part of the taxable year, complete Schedules B and C on page 2 of Form IT-214, using the instructions below. Add 25 percent of your adjusted rent paid (from Schedule C) to the prorated part of any charges you list on Schedule B. Enter this total on line 7.

Schedule B

Enter on lines 25 and 26 any county, city, town, village or school district taxes and assessments that you and all qualified members of your household paid during 1982 (do not include penalty and interest charges). For persons 65 or older, enter on line 27 the amount exempted from taxation under Section 467 of the Real Property Tax Law. Add lines 25 through 27 and enter the total on line 28. Transfer this amount to line 7 on page 1.

Schedule C

If your 1982 rent payments included charges for heat, gas, electricity, furnishings or board which were not separately stated, complete lines 29 through 32. Enter on line 29 the total rent you and all other members of your household paid; do not include any subsidized part of your rental charge. Figure the amounts to be entered on lines 30, 31 and 32. Transfer the amount on line 32 to line 7 on page 1.

If your 1982 rent payments did not include charges for heat, gas, electricity, furnishings or board or if rental charges were separately stated, complete lines 33 and 34 of Schedule C. Enter on line 33 the amount of rent paid, not counting charges for heat, gas, electricity, furnishings, board or any subsidized part of your rental charge. Figure the amount to be entered on line 34 and transfer it to line 7 on page 1.

If your adjusted rent (line 31 or line 33) is more than $300 per month, **stop**; you do not qualify for this credit.

Line 8

Household Gross Income

Before figuring your household gross income, enter the names and social security numbers of all members of your household, including yourself, on page 2, Schedule D. Also give the age of any **qualified** household member who was 65 or older as of December 31, 1982. If you need more space, list additional names on a separate sheet and attach it to Form IT-214.

Figure your entry for line 8 (household gross income) on **Schedule A,** page 2 of Form IT-214. Enter on line 15 the number of household members listed in Schedule D. Enter on line 16 the total federal adjusted gross income of you and all members of your household. If you or any member of your household do not have to file a federal return, include the amount that would be included in federal adjusted gross income if a federal return had been required.

Enter on line 17 the total additions to federal adjusted gross income required by Section 612(b) of the Tax Law. For a list of these additions, see Publication 308, *Real Property Tax Credit,* or page 14 of the instructions for Form IT-201. Include the total of these additions that apply to you and all members of your household, even if a New York State income tax return is not required.

Enter on lines 18 through 23 the total of each type of income you and all members of your household received during 1982.

If someone was a member of your household for only part of the taxable year, include on lines 16 through 23 the income he received while he was a member of your household.

Add lines 16 through 23 and enter the total on line 24. Round this amount to the nearest whole dollar and transfer it to line 8 on page 1. If this amount is more than $16,000, **stop**; you do not qualify for the credit.

Line 9 Rate

Using the table following line 9, find the rate that applies to your household gross income and enter it on line 9.

Line 10

Multiply the amount on line 8 by the rate on line 9 and enter the result on line 10.

Line 11

Subtract line 10 from line 7 and enter the difference on line 11. If the amount on line 10 is more than the amount on line 7, **stop**; no credit is allowed.

Lines 12 and 13

Follow the instructions on Form IT-214, lines 12 and 13, to find your entry for those lines.

Line 14

Real Property Tax Credit

The real property tax credit for your household is the amount on line 12 or line 13 — whichever is less. Enter the lesser amount on line 14.

If more than one member of your household is filing Form IT-214, divide the line 14 amount equally among all filers. You can divide the line 14 amount any way you want if you each agree to the amount of your share and attach a copy of the agreement to your Form IT-214. Enter only your share of the line 14 amount on your Form IT-214 (and on your return if you have to file one).

If you are married and filing a joint return, you do not have to divide the credit.

If you are filing a 1982 New York State income tax return, transfer your line 14 amount to Form IT-200, line 14 or Form IT-201, line 20. If any qualified member of your household, including yourself, is 65 or older, check the box on line 14 of Form IT-200 or on line 20 of Form IT-201.

Your credit will be subtracted from the amount of tax you owe. Any amount over the tax you owe will be refunded to you. **Sign Form IT-214 and attach it to the return you are filing.**

If you are not filing a 1982 New York State income tax return, sign and date Form IT-214 and mail it to:

New York State Income Tax
State Campus
Albany, NY 12227

Your real property tax credit payment will be mailed to you.

Your Legal Rights When You Rent a Room

prepared by Gerry Careccia, Ettie Taichman, and Hal Bishop

illustrations by Susan Anderson

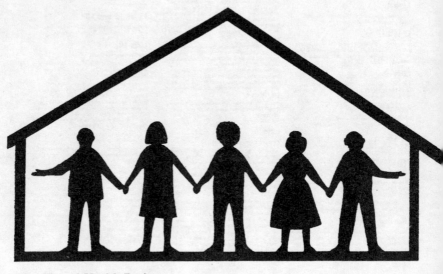

The Mental Health Project
School of Social Welfare
State University of New York at Stony Brook
Long Island, New York 11794
Stephen M. Rose
Project Director
1980

This booklet is for you if you rent a room in a . . .

rooming house,
boarding house,
residential hotel, motel, or
a one or two family house.

People who rent rooms have legal rights
although those rights are not always widely known.
When you rent a room you are a tenant
and you are protected by the law.
You have the right, for example, to a place
which is safe and reasonably clean and comfortable.

And, of course, when you rent a room
you have the same political and personal rights as everyone else.
You have . . .
   the right to manage your own affairs,
   the right to make your own decisions,
   the right to fair and decent treatment,
   and so on.
And like every other member of the community,
you are entitled to dignity, to respect and to equal protection
of the law.

Unfortunately, information about the laws which may protect you
is often difficult to get.
That is why this booklet was written.
Your Legal Rights When You Rent a Room was written to inform you
of some of the rights you have . . .
   as a tenant,
   as a citizen,
   and as a member of the community.

We hope you will find it useful.

When you rent a room
you enter into a business agreement with your landlord.

You pay rent.
In turn, your landlord provides certain services.

Both you and your landlord have an interest in knowing
what is expected.
Both of you want to know what you will be paying.
And both want to know *exactly* what you will be receiving.

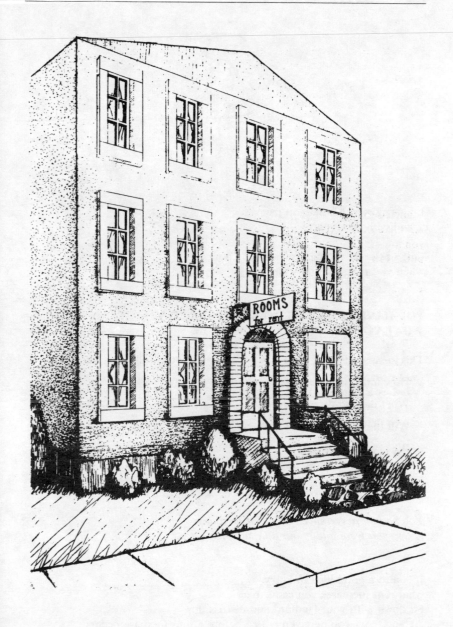

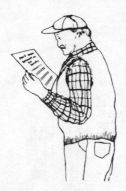

Let's begin with what you pay . . .
    and with how you pay it.

One of the first things you should know
when you rent a room is that

**YOU HAVE THE RIGHT TO KNOW EXACTLY
WHAT YOUR RENTAL COSTS WILL BE.**

This means it is your right to have answers to the following questions:

How much is my rent each month? $ ....

What day is my rent due?   ....

Will there be any extra charges?   ....

What will cost extra?

    .... $ ....
    .... $ ....
    .... $ ....

*You should never have to pay for anything
unless you were told about it in advance.*

It is also a good idea to know
what rent increases you can expect.
Sit down with your landlord and discuss this.
Arrange that you be given notice before a rent increase occurs.
And ask your landlord if he or she can tell you
when your rent will be increased – and by how much.

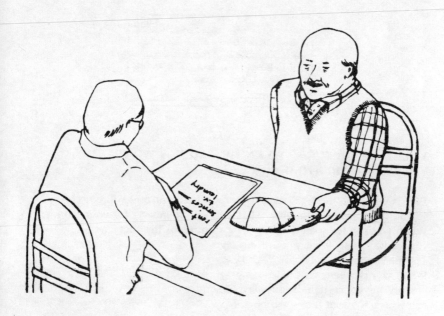

Ask . . .

When is my rent likely to be raised? ....

How much will my rent be? ....

Will I get any notice before my rent is raised? ....

How much notice? ....

You can also ask your landlord for a receipt.

YOU HAVE THE RIGHT TO A RECEIPT WHEN YOU PAY YOUR RENT.

When you pay for something you are entitled to a receipt.
A receipt is a written record of . . .
    how much you paid,
    when you paid, and
    what you get for your money.

A receipt helps you to keep a record of your expenses.
It makes good sense to keep track of your business dealings this way.

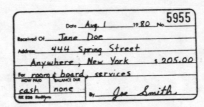

YOU HAVE THE RIGHT TO KNOW EXACTLY WHAT YOU WILL BE RENTING.

Just as you have the legal right to know what your rent will be,
so you have the right to know what you will be getting for your money.
When you pay for something, like cigarettes, for instance,
you know exactly what you are buying.
The same should apply with your rent.
When you pay your rent,
you are buying certain conditions and services.
Know exactly what those will be.

This sounds easy.
It isn't always that simple.
See if you know what you are getting for your rent.
Check to see if you can answer all the questions on the next two pages.

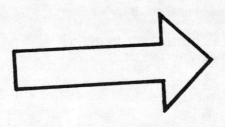

Information Sheet about the New Rooming House/Residential Tenant Rights Law

(Chapter 739 of the Laws of 1982) Real Property Actions and Proceedings Law §711 (as amended August 1982)

Prepared By Diane Johnson, CSW

Legal Advocacy Project
School of Social Welfare, SUNY, Stony Brook, N.Y.

with the help of Mental Health Law Project
Nassau/Suffolk Law Services Committee, Bay Shore, N.Y.

What follows is a series of questions and answers concerning the rooming house/residential hotel tenant rights law passed by the New York State Legislature in August 1982. We have attempted to explain as simply as possible those rights, entitlements, protections and strategies which are now available, as a result of this law, to residents living in these settings.

Be advised that this information is not offered as a substitute for seeking legal advice. It is, however, meant to offer information to advocates and to their clients living in rooming houses and residential hotels and to suggest strategies for ensuring that people's rights as tenants are not violated.

We want to stress the importance of using this law – otherwise, the changes it has enacted will be meaningless. It is important that rooming house and residential hotel tenants know of their new rights and protections, that they insist on being granted these rights and that advocates take an informed stance in pursuing any violations of these guaranteed rights and entitlements.

Prospective plaintiffs must be encouraged and supported through what in many situations will be a long, hard and potentially threatening struggle.

Central to this struggle will be the necessity for the plaintiff to have the information necessary to make informed choices throughout the process. Support must include the joining together by the plaintiff of as many resource agencies and people as possible.

We would be interested in any reactions to this Information Sheet and would welcome your thoughts and suggestions for improving its usefulness. Call us at (516) 444-3174.

Questions and Answers About the New Rooming House/Residential Hotel Tenant Rights Law

(Chapter 739 of the Laws of 1982)
Real Property Actions and Proceedings Law §711
(as amended August 1982)

Q. What does this law do?
A. It grants 'tenant' status to anyone who lives for thirty consecutive days or more in a rooming house or residential hotel (excluding a transient occupant), and it allows the person to seek redress through the courts for any infringement of his or her rights as a tenant.
Q. What is so important about this law?
A. When you talk about the law pertaining to rental housing, basically there are two categories of people: owners and tenants. Until the passage of this law, residents of rooming houses and residential hotels were considered to be neither owners nor tenants (they were considered 'transients') and consequently they did not have any of the rights that other tenants have. Because this law gives rooming house and residential hotel dwellers 'tenant' status, it entitles them to the same rights and protections that all other tenants have.
Q. What rights does a 'tenant' have?
A. Many, including:
  – the protection against immediate and/or 'self-help' eviction (a tenant must be given 'timely and adequate' notice before having to vacate).
  – the guarantee that the premises rented will be fit for human habitation.
  – the guarantee that the premises rented will be free from conditions which endanger life, health or safety.
  – the protection against retaliatory eviction for complaints about housing code violations or about the landlord's failure to obey the lease.
  – the protection of having a day in court if any of these tenant rights are violated.
Q. What is a 'self-help' eviction?
A. A 'self-help' eviction is one in which the landlord forces the tenant out, either through the use of physical force or through the use of threats. An

example of a 'self-help' eviction would be a case where the landlord plugs or changes the lock to the tenant's room in order to keep the tenant out. Another example of a 'self-help' eviction would be a case where the landlord threatens the tenant with bodily harm if the tenant does not vacate immediately.

Q. When you are talking about protection against immediate eviction, what does 'timely and adequate' notice to vacate mean?

A. The courts have held that 'timely and adequate' notice varies according to how often a person pays rent. For example, a person who pays rent weekly is considered to have a week-to-week tenancy and is entitled to seven days notice to vacate *from the time his or her next rent payment is due*. A person who pays rent monthly is entitled to thirty or thirty-one days notice to vacate (depending upon the month), *the thirty (or thirty-one) days commencing from the time the next payment is due*.

Q. Do you mean that a landlord might actually have to give a week-to-week tenant more than seven days notice to vacate or might have to give a month-to-month tenant more than thirty (or thirty-one) days notice to vacate?

A. Yes. For example, if a person who is a month-to-month tenant paying rent on the 1st of the month receives notice to vacate on the 10th of the month, s/he is entitled to remain in residence the rest of the month during which s/he received notice (from the 11th to the 31st) and *all* of the next month.

Q. If a person is a week-to-week tenant, how would this process work?

A. If a week-to-week tenant pays rent every Monday and then receives notice to vacate on a Wednesday, s/he is entitled to remain in residence the rest of that week (Wednesday through Sunday) and *all* of the following week.

Q. Does a tenant have to receive the notice to vacate in writing?

A. No, oral notice can be given, but landlords are always advised that written notice is better because then there is less question that notice was given. Of course, the landlord must still prove, if s/he has to go to court, that the written notice was actually given.

Q. Does this law mean that a landlord has to go to court to evict a tenant ('. . . he shall not be removed from possession except in a special proceeding.')?

A. No. A landlord must go to court to evict someone only if a tenant refuses to vacate the premises after the required amount of notice has been given (for example, thirty or thirty-one days for a month-to-month tenancy, seven days for a week-to-week tenancy, etc. – see the questions above) or if the landlord wishes to evict the tenant because of a breach of the terms of the lease.

Q. If a landlord does go to court to bring an eviction proceeding against a tenant, how long does this process take?

A. The law states that when a landlord goes to court to initiate an eviction proceeding (known as a 'summary proceeding'), such a proceeding shall take place *not sooner than five days* and *not more than twelve days* after the action was initiated. The action is initiated when the necessary court papers are prepared, served on the tenant and filed in court by the landlord.

Q. Suppose the landlord says someone is an 'objectionable' tenant. Can the landlord evict the person without giving the proper amount of notice?

A. The answer to this question is rather complicated and has several parts: First, if the tenant has a *written* lease:

- a written lease for a fixed period of time (for example, one month, one year, etc.) can only be terminated by the landlord before it expires in case of *breach of its terms*.
- in order for a written lease to be terminated because of 'objectionable' behavior, the lease must include a statement to the effect that 'good behavior' is required and that 'objectionable' behavior constitutes a breach of the lease.
- if a written lease *does not* contain a 'good behavior' clause, a tenant *cannot* be evicted for 'objectionable' behavior.

   (Note: most landlords use a standard lease, the type available in stationery stores, which *does* contain a 'good behavior' clause.)

If a landlord wishes to evict a tenant for 'objectionable' behavior and the tenant has signed a lease containing a 'good behavior' clause, the landlord still must go to court to remove the tenant. Before the courts allow such an eviction, they will want to be certain that the tenant's behavior is significantly 'objectionable.' It is important to remember that the law is very specific about who constitutes an 'objectionable' tenant. In general, an 'objectionable' tenant:

- is someone who is engaged in criminal activity (for example, selling drugs or engaging in prostitution).
- is someone whose use of the property is unwarranted or unreasonable causing annoyance, inconvenience, discomfort or damage to others.

However, there are two important points to keep in mind regarding 'objectionability':

- mere annoyances in and of themselves *do not* make a tenant 'undesirable' or 'objectionable.'
- 'undesirability' or 'objectionability' involves the idea of *continuing or recurring action*. In other words, the 'objectionable' behavior must have continued over a period of time.

It is unlikely, therefore, that a court would declare a tenant 'objectionable' who, for example, talks to him or herself or who engages in other behavior not viewed as 'normal', *as long as that behavior does not hurt others*. On the other hand, a tenant who stockpiles garbage in his or her room would, in all likelihood, be declared 'objectionable' if the landlord can show that such behavior *has continued over a period of time* and is not a one-time occurrence.*

Q. Continuing with the previous question, if the courts do find a particular tenant to be 'objectionable,' how soon can s/he be evicted?

A. There may be variations in actual time from region to region, but often the courts will stay (hold up) the eviction for a short while if the tenant has a good reason for such a delay. Needing additional time to find other housing is a good reason for granting such a stay. Therefore, tenants should always argue for additional time. Even in those cases where the court grants the landlord the right to remove the tenant 'immediately,' the tenant does not have to vacate until served with papers by the sheriff, constable, etc. After these papers have been served, the tenant still has 72 hours before having to vacate.

Q. What happens if the tenant does not have a written lease, but has an *oral* lease? Do the same procedures apply?

A. If the tenant has an *oral* lease, the following conditions hold:
  – an oral lease can be terminated by the landlord *at any time for no stated reason*. In other words, the landlord does not have to find a reason to break the lease (such as 'objectionable' behavior) but can simply tell the tenant that s/he must move. There is no court proceeding required in this type of situation.
  – when the landlord terminates an oral lease for no stated reason, the tenant *must still be given the proper amount of notice*. As we have explained previously, the proper amount of time would be *at least* seven days for a week-to-week tenant and *at least* thirty or thirty-one days for a month-to-month tenant.
  – an oral lease can also be terminated by the landlord if the tenant breaks the terms of the lease (for example, not paying his or her rent on time). In such a case, if the tenant refuses to move out, the landlord *must* go to court and commence a legal proceeding to remove the tenant. Such a proceeding is called a 'summary' proceeding. It is important to remember that the landlord is *not* permitted to use force or threats to get the tenant to move out *even if the tenant has broken the terms of the lease*.

Q. Are you saying that this law prohibits 'self-help' evictions – that even if the tenant breaks the terms of the lease, the landlord cannot force the tenant out, either with threats or with physical force?

A. We believe the answer is yes. If the tenant breaks the terms of the lease (either oral or written) and the tenant refuses to move, the landlord *must* go to court and bring a legal proceeding (summary proceeding) against the tenant. This procedure protects the tenant against 'self-help' evictions and guarantees the tenant the right to present his or her side of the story to

---

* see Real Property Actions and Proceedings Law (RPAPL), §711(5) and Notes 92 and 121–40 for a more detailed explanation.

the court. If the court finds the landlord's eviction proceeding to be justified (for example, the rent was not paid and there was no excuse for non-payment), a warrant will be issued by the court and served on the tenant by the sheriff, marshall or constable. After the warrant has been served, the tenant will have 72 hours to vacate.

Q. What happens if a landlord does lock-out a tenant or force the tenant out with threats?

A. As we have stated above, it is against the law for a landlord to evict a tenant without a court order (a warrant served by a sheriff, marshall or constable). If a tenant is evicted or locked-out without this court order, the tenant may do several things:
- if the landlord has retained the tenant's possessions, s/he can file criminal charges against the landlord (for larceny).
- the tenant may go into Supreme Court and seek an injunction placing him or her back in the premises.
- if the tenant does not return to the premises, s/he may sue the landlord in Small Claims Court for rebate of the unused portion of the rent, for rebate of his or her security deposit and for the return of the value of his or her belongings.
- the tenant may add to his or her civil suit a claim for treble (triple) damages for unlawful eviction if the eviction was done in a forcible manner or in a way that put the tenant in fear of personal violence. (see RPAPL §853)
- the tenant may also re-enter the premises to recover possession of his or her rented space and/or belongings as long as s/he does not disturb the peace or destroy or damage property. Police can sometimes be called upon to help a tenant recover his or her personal belongings, but will usually not help someone recover possession of his or her rented space.

Q. If a tenant and a landlord agree to some sort of leasetype agreement, can certain provisions in this lease supercede the provisions of this law? For example, can a person waive his or her right to 'timely and adequate' notice to vacate?

A. This is uncertain. Real Property Law, §235-C permits the courts to declare all or any part of a lease 'unconscionable' and to decline to enforce it. In general, 'unconscionable' means any lease provision which unreasonably restricts the liberty of the tenant or is overly repressive. It could be argued that a provision whereby a tenant waives his or her right to 'timely and adequate' notice is unconscionable. However, there have been certain limited instances in which the courts have upheld lease provisions which allow the landlord to give 'short notice' (for example, less than seven days for a week-to-week tenancy, less than thirty or thirty-one days for a month-to-month tenancy). These instances have been few, but it is wise to advise tenants not to agree to a lease with a 'short notice' provision.

Q. Does this law mean that a person living in a rooming house or residential hotel is entitled to a written lease or rental agreement if s/he asks for one?

A. No. A landlord does not have to give a tenant a written lease. However, if there is no written lease, it is assumed that an oral lease covering such things as amount of rent, when it shall be paid, etc., is in effect.

Q. Because of this law, all tenants now have certain '*warranty of habitability*' protections. What does this mean?

A. According to Real Property Law, §235–b, every landlord guarantees that his or her rental property is:
   – fit for human habitation
   – free from conditions dangerous or detrimental to the life, health or safety of the occupants.

The landlord further guarantees that the premises will be maintained in this manner. *A tenant cannot waive or agree to modification of this right to a habitable premises.*

Q. Can a tenant refuse to pay all or part of the rent if a landlord does not maintain the premises so that it is fit for human habitation or free from conditions endangering the health or safety of the tenants?

A. Yes, a tenant may withhold all or part of the rent, but before doing so s/he is advised to seek legal advise to ensure that all of the correct procedures are followed. In general:
   – the tenant must first ask the landlord to fix any dangerous conditions (if possible, this should be done *in writing* and the tenant should be sure to keep a copy of the letter).
   – the tenant must also report these dangerous conditions to the local health or building department (again, if possible, in writing, keeping a copy of the letter).

It is crucial that the tenant, then, hold onto the rent money to deposit it with the court if and when the landlord starts an eviction proceeding for non-payment of rent. If the landlord fails to make the repairs in a reasonable amount of time and then brings an eviction proceeding, the tenant may raise the landlord's 'warranty of habitability' obligation as a defense and ask for a reduction in the amount owed the landlord.

Q. What would be some examples of situations in which a tenant could withhold rent on the ground that living conditions posed a threat to his or her health or safety?

A. Of course, there are many situations which could exist which would be unique to individual dwellings, but in general, any time there is a *lack of heat, running water, light, electricity, adequate sewage facilities* or *infestation by rodents*, a strong argument can be made that health and/or safety endangering conditions exist. In addition, there are numerous structural problems (for example, a broken main staircase, ceilings falling in, a roof that leaks substantially, causing tenants' rooms to be flooded, etc.) which could also be cited as endangering a tenant's health and/or safety. As we have stated above, a tenant would be wise to seek legal advise to ensure that the situation is sufficiently dangerous to justify, in the eyes of the court, the withholding of rent by the tenant.

Q. Is there anything other than withholding the rent that a tenant can do to force the landlord to make needed repairs?

A. Yes, there are several other things which can be done. Real Property Actions and Proceedings Law (RPAPL), Article 7–A allows tenants of multiple dwellings (rooming houses, residential hotels and SRO's are all multiple dwellings) in *New York City, Nassau, Suffolk, Rockland* and *Westchester* Counties (these counties only) to bring court actions against landlords to correct life, health and safety endangering conditions. Such actions can be brought if:
   – one-third or more of the tenants in the building agree to the action
   – the existing situation is clearly a threat to the life, health or safety of the tenants (see the previous question)
   – the situation posing a threat to the life, health or safety of the tenants *has existed for five days*
   (Note: As we understand it, the five days *do not* have to be consecutive. As long as the dangerous situation has existed on five separate occasions, we believe that there is a cause for action.)

   If the courts decide in favor of the tenant, that is, that a dangerous situation exists, it can order that all rent be paid to a court-appointed administrator. The court will then direct the administrator to make the needed repairs. After the repair work is done, the landlord will then be allowed to collect the rent again.

Q. What about tenants who live outside the greater New York area – is there anything other than withholding the rent which they can do?

A. Yes. Any tenant (regardless of the county in which s/he lives) can take action to ensure that serious, safety, health or life-threatening conditions get corrected. If a tenant chooses this course of action, s/he *must* be sure to follow certain procedures:
   – the tenant must first have asked the landlord to correct the dangerous situation (in writing with the tenant keeping a copy of the letter).
   – the tenant must also have reported these dangerous conditions to the local health and/or building departments (in writing, keeping a copy of the letter).
   – *the landlord must have been given a reasonable amount of time to repair the dangerous condition.*

   If all of these procedures have been followed, the tenant can, if s/he chooses, make arrangements to have the condition repaired and deduct the cost of such repairs from his or her rent payment. However the tenant is cautioned to remember:
   – to keep all receipts for any repair work done in case the matter eventually ends up in court.

- all repair work that is done must be done at a 'reasonable' cost.
- it would be unwise to undertake having any major repair work done.
- this 'repair and deduct' strategy can only be used *if the procedures outlined previously have been followed and if the condition poses a serious threat to the tenant's life, health or safety.*

Q. What is the role of the Department of Social Services in relation to the 'warranty of habitability' obligation of landlords?

A. According to Social Services Law, §143–b, in cases where recipients are in 'restricted payment' status (that is, the Department of Social Services is paying their rent for them directly to the landlord), a local Department of Social Services (DSS) has the right to withhold the rent allowance *in cases where housing conditions violate health or housing codes or are dangerous to life, health or safety of the occupants.*

Q. If DSS does withhold a recipient's rent payment because unsafe housing conditions exist, won't the tenant be evicted?

A. If DSS follows this course of action, the landlord may choose to initiate an eviction proceeding (in order to immediately evict the tenant) or the landlord may simply give the tenant the required amount of notice that the lease is being terminated (seven days for a week-to-week tenant, thirty of thirty-one days for a month-to-month tenant). However, if either of these actions happen, the tenant is guaranteed certain protections:
- in the case of an eviction proceeding brought by the landlord, the non-payment of the rent by DSS is an *automatic defence* for the tenant. The burden of proof then is on the landlord to prove that the dangerous conditions have been corrected and that s/he is entitled to once again receive rent payments.
- if the tenant is given notice that the lease is being terminated, the tenant can refuse to move. Such an action will force the landlord to initiate a court proceeding to remove him or her. During this proceeding, the tenant can claim 'retaliatory eviction' – that s/he is being evicted for reporting a violation of existing codes, rules and/or regulations.

Q. How can a tenant or his or her advocate go about getting the Department of Social Services to use this rent-withholding strategy?

A. As we have previously mentioned, the tenant must begin by notifying the landlord of any serious health, safety or life-threatening conditions which needed correcting. (Remember, do this notification in writing, if possible and keep a copy). If the landlord does not correct the problem(s), the tenant should then notify the local Health and/or Building Departments about the existence of violations to their codes (again, preferably in writing). The tenant should indicate to these officials that s/he is a recipient of DSS funds. Upon receipt of such a letter, the Health and/or Building Departments are supposed to inspect the premises to check for the alleged violations. If the tenant's claims are verified, the Health and/or Building inspectors are then supposed to notify the Local Welfare

District to withhold payment of rent until such time as the cited violations are corrected. At this time, it is also a good idea for the tenant and/or his or her advocate to notify the Department of Social Services about the violations and to request that the rent not be paid until the violations are corrected. Again, remember that this strategy can only be used for those tenants whose rent is paid directly to the landlord.

Q. Getting back to the issue of 'retaliatory eviction' – how does a tenant prove 'retaliatory eviction'?

A. At the risk of sounding like a broken record, we repeat that it is very important that a tenant *keep a record in writing if possible, of all complaints filed with the landlord, the health department, the local building department, Department of Social Services, etc.* If the tenant is unable to make the complaints in writing and does so orally, s/he should still be sure to keep a record of the conversations, who was spoken to, what was discussed, what course of action was agreed upon, etc. If the tenant is subsequently evicted for reporting violations, this documentation will be very important in substantiating the tenant's claim of 'retaliatory eviction'.

Q. Are the people who live in places know as 'Veterans' Homes' considered to be tenants under this law?

A. Even though veterans' homes are under the control of the Veteran's Administration, we believe that they are similar to boarding homes, rooming houses and residential hotels in that they are set up primarily to provide room and board to the people living there. We believe, therefore, that residents of veterans' homes are considered under this law to be 'tenants'.

Q. Is someone who has lived in emergency housing supplied by the Department of Social Services for more than thirty days (at one location) now considered to be a 'tenant'?

A. We do not know the answer to this question, but would argue 'yes'. Even though the law specifically excludes 'transient occupants', the Department of Social Services has been known to house homeless people in 'emergency' housing on a more long-term, permanent basis. In these types of cases, we would argue that the people should be considered 'tenants' with all of the ensuing rights and protections.

The following is the text of Chapter Law 739 of the Laws of 1982 as it amends Real Property Actions and Proceedings Law, §711.* It is because this law

---

* As soon as the next *McKinney's Consolidated Laws of New York Pocket Part* is issued, this law will be known as Real Property Actions and Proceedings Law, §711 as amended, August 1982.

specifically grants 'tenant' status to rooming house and hotel occupants that these people (provided that they have been in residence for thirty consecutive days or longer) are entitled to all of the rights and protections which we have outlined in this Information Sheet.

Laws of New York

Eviction from Lodgings – Certain Occupants of Rooming Houses or Hotels

Chapter 739
Approved 27 July 1982, effective as provided in section 2

AN ACT to amend the real property actions and proceedings law, in relation to evictions from lodgings

The People of the State of New York, represented in Senate and Assembly, do enact as follows:

Section 1. The section heading and opening paragraph of section seven hundred eleven of the real property actions and proceedings law, as added by chapter three hundred twelve of the laws of nineteen hundred sixty-two, is amended to read as follows:

Grounds where landlord-tenant relationship exist.

A tenant shall include an occupant of one or more rooms in a rooming house or a resident not including a transient occupant, of one or more rooms in a hotel who has been in possession for thirty consecutive days or longer; he shall not be removed from possession except in a special proceeding. A special proceeding may be maintained under this article upon the following grounds: (the rest of the existing law remains the same – see RPAPL, Section 711).

Section 2. This act shall take effect on the thirtieth day after it shall have become law.

The underlined material indicates changes brought about by this law. The text above is the law as it now reads.

Important Aspects of the Adult Home Access Law: Chapter 843 of the Laws of 1983

1 Adult Homes may *not* restrict access or interfere with confidential visits with residents by:
   – family members
   – friends
   – legal representatives
   – legal counsels
   – case managers
   – community organizations or service agencies providing a *free* service or *educational* program to residents
   – not-for-profit agencies, service organizations or associations which visit to help residents *secure needed services* and *resolve problems* concerning their care and treatment.
   NOTE: This law *guarantees* access to these individuals and groups. It should not be interpreted to *restrict* access of others!

2 The right to determine whom s/he will see is that of the resident:
   – a resident has the right to deny any visit
   – a resident has a right to terminate any visit at any time.

3 Denial of access to any of the individuals or groups listed above by the adult homeowner can only take place if:
   – the operator has 'reasonable cause' to believe that such an individual would 'directly endanger' the safety of the residents.

4 The following procedures for visiting residents in their rooms must be followed:
   – all visitors guaranteed access must identify themselves to the resident before entering a resident's room
   – all visitors must state the purpose of the visit to the resident
   – before entering a resident's room, all visitors must receive the permission of the resident and the resident's roommate
   – a visitor does not have to have the adult homeowner or manager announce his or her visit.

5 Visits with residents may take place in a resident's room if the above procedures are followed or may take place in a common area which the operator must make available for such visits.

6 Adult homes must be open for visits with residents for a period of at least *ten hours* between 9 a.m. and 8 p.m.
   – hours may be extended by agreement with the home.

7 The only other restriction on services providers is:
   – In order to be guaranteed access, not-for-profit corporations, community organizations and associations (in other words, all those who do not fit under the categories of family members, friends, legal representatives, legal counsels, or case managers mentioned in 1 above) must file a copy of their certificate of incorporation or their bylaws with the State Department of Social Services.
   – Address to send papers to: Corinne Plummer, Deputy Commissioner, Department of Social Services, Division of Adult Services, 40 N. Pearl St., Albany, N.Y. 12243.

8 If an individual or group is denied access, the operator must:
   – record a detailed written statement describing the reasons for denial of access
   – make this statement accessible to residents and the groups denied access.

9 A person denied access may regain access by:
   – bringing an action in Supreme Court for an order granting access.

10 Penalties for denial of access:
   – If the Supreme Court finds that denial of access was done in 'bad faith', the operator shall be liable for:
     – all costs, including reasonable attorney's fees
     – a civil penalty not to exceed $50 a day for each day access was denied, to be awarded at the discretion of the court

11 For a complete text of the law, see New York State Social Services Law §461–a(3) (b), when the new pocketpart is printed.

FOR FURTHER INFORMATION OR QUESTIONS CONTACT:

Diane Johnson
Legal Advocacy Project
School of Social Welfare
S.U.N.Y. at Stony Brook
Stony Brook, N.Y. 11794
(516) 444–3174

Candace Scott Appleton
The Mental Health Law
   Project
28 Park Avenue
Bay Shore, N.Y. 11706
(516) 665–2000

Comments on Division of Adult Services Proposed Amendments Governing Adult Homes

Prepared by:

Diane Johnson, Mental Health Project
S.U.N.Y. at Stony Brook

Paul Sivak, Sayville Project
Community Support Services Program

Jan Milthaler, Sayville Project
Community Support Services Program

February 1984

Comments on newly proposed DAS regulations

We would like to take this opportunity to comment on the newly proposed regulations of the Division of Adult Services for private proprietary homes for adults. The focus of our remarks will be the effect these proposed changes in regulation will have on the quality of life available to people living in private proprietary facilities.

Before addressing any specific regulatory proposals, there are several overriding issues. First, nowhere in the new regulations does the Department* clarify the status of adult home resident vis-à-vis the adult home operator. There is an assumption underlying all of the regulations that the adult home operator is the implicit head of a 'treatment team' whose job it is to help residents with an array of psychiatric, social and adjustment problems. This is

---

* 'Department' in this paper shall be meant to refer to the NYS Department of Social Services.

a false assumption. On the contrary, there exists a contractual landlord-tenant-like relationship** between the adult home operator and each adult home resident. The operators and staff of the profit-based adult homes are *not* mental health service providers, but are business people providing housing and 'personal care' services to residents of these facilities in exchange for profit. Any regulations purporting to govern adult residential care facilities, if they are truly intended to protect the interests and serve the needs of those people living in these facilities, must recognize this relationship and must state explicitly the contractual nature of such a relationship.

Directly related to the existence of this legally constituted relationship between adult home operator and adult home resident is a second related matter: as tenants and as citizens of the communities in which they reside, adult home residents must be free to choose which services they wish to use from any available to them as part of their contractual agreements with the operators. Further, residents must be free to negotiate any additional or alternative services in the community at large, for example, using a doctor other than the 'house doctor,' which they deem to be in their own best interests. This perspective requires that the Department word any regulations pertaining to services in such a way as to indicate that the adult home operator is obligated to offer certain in-house services as part of the admission agreement, but that the resident is not confined to using *only* these offered services. The final *choice* lies with the adult home resident in determining which services she/he wishes to use. It must be stated clearly that the resident has the right, just as any other citizen does, to determine *what* health, mental health and social services she/he needs and *from whom* she/he wishes to receive these services.

There is a final general point which we wish to make. The new regulations stipulate that in-house case management services must be provided, either by the adult home operator (in facilities with less than fifty residents) or by a case manager employed specifically for that purpose by the operator (in facilities with more than fifty residents). This regulation fails to recognize the conflict of interest inherent in any contractual, profit-based service relationship. Further, it presumes that the needs of adult home residents are most often the same as those of the operators or exist independently from them, that is, are unrelated to conditions in the home. It presumes that when the needs of operator and resident conflict, such a conflict can be resolved to everyone's satisfaction by a house-employed case manager. This is a false assumption and one which we will address at length in the course of our remarks.

** Given that Social Service Law provides protection to adult home residents similar to those offered to tenants under Landlord-Tenant Law (for example, due process protection, specific eviction procedures, notice of intent to increase rent, etc.), we have chosen to describe the adult home operator-resident relationship as a 'landlord-tenant like' relationship.

At this point, we would like to elaborate in more detail the three general points made above: (1) that the relationship between adult home operator and adult home resident is similar to that of landlord and tenant, not that of health care professional and patient; (2) that the adult home resident must be free to choose which services she/he wishes to use from the array offered by the adult home operator and must be free to make other service arrangements as she/he so desires; and (3) that there is a built-in conflict of interest situation which exists and *can never be overcome* when in-house case managers are employed to provide case management services to adult home residents.

First, let us discuss the notion of adult home operator as a mental health 'treatment team' member. Private proprietary homes for adults are *not* treatment facilities nor were they ever meant to be. They are not licensed or designated by the Office of Mental Health as treatment facilities. Historically, such residences have provided housing for the physically disabled, frail elderly who were unable to live independently. When deinstitutionalization became the policy of the state, many former psychiatric patients found themselves placed in adult homes, not because these homes could provide treatment in the community or were even a proper level of care, but because there were no other housing options sought by discharging hospitals.*

In recognition of the fact that many psychiatric patients have been placed in adult homes during the past twenty years, regulations were adopted in 1978 which delineated a role for the Office of Mental Health in relation to proposing additional regulations presumed to be necessary for the protection of their clients residing in adult homes. However, to our knowledge, the Office of Mental Health has not chosen to exercise this prerogative, acting instead to leave the regulation of these homes to the Department of Social Services. Joint Office of Mental Health-Department of Social Services inspection teams have been functioning for several years, but the Office of Mental Health participant has neither a specified role or grievance mechanism, particularly in cases of actual or potential disputes with the Department of Social Services inspector on whose turf the action is taking place. While Office of Mental Health policy regards adult homes as significantly outside the domain of their Department, in no way does it regard the operators or the staffs of such residences as a formal part of any mental health 'treatment team.' Furthermore, because of its reluctance to assume adequate care in these facilities, the Office of Mental Health requires owners to have some form of contract with a mental health service provider in the community.

It is easy to see why confusion exists around the belief that the adult home operator is a 'treatment team' member. Indeed, the existing Division of Adult

---

* Indeed, as the 1977 report of The Hynes Commission stated, many mental health workers came to realize the inappropriateness of the adult home placements, conceding the 'fundamental disparity' between the kind of care, supervision and support needed by many dischargees and the kind of care and services provided by adult homes (pp. 30–1).

Services regulations and proposed new regulations do much to confuse and obscure the issue because the nature of the relationship between operator and resident is never clearly delineated. The proprietor of the home, in exchange for payment, is providing the resident with room, board and certain specified services. Because some of the services which both the old and newly proposed regulations require of the operators are mental health-like services, the issue of the actual relationship between adult home operator and resident often becomes clouded. For example, the regulations require that facilities with 25 per cent or more mentally disabled persons released or discharged from Office of Mental Health facilities contract out for mental health services with a nearby state psychiatric clinic or other appropriate service provider (487.7 (b)). This is an important regulation obviously meant to help ensure that former psychiatric clients have *access* to sometimes needed mental health care (although this regulation simultaneously maintains a lack of choice by residents over their care). However, this regulation *in no way* implies that the operator of the adult home is to provide these services; that the operator is a qualified mental health professional; or that the operator and the adult home staff are part of any mental health 'treatment team.'

The basic profit or business-centered, contractual relationship between operator and resident is further obscured when one looks at the particular regulations which have to do with the qualifications required of staff members. Under the proposed new regulations, those individuals to be employed as 'case managers' must have training in human resources or service delivery and must have experience working with a dependent population (487.9 (d) (4)). Adult home administrators are required also to have certain educational training and work experience, one area of which *may be* (but does not have to be) human services or social work. Thus, the regulations help to foster the idea that adult residential care facility staff members as well as the operators are mental health professionals. We want to emphasize one point: having a case manager on the staff of an adult home or an operator who has training and experience working with an adult dependent population *does not* de facto make those individuals or that particular home part of any 'treatment team' which may be envisioned as providing proper or adequate follow-up care in the uncomprised interests of clients discharged from the state hospital system into the community.

At this point, it is important to note that our intent is not to be critical of the human service or social work training required of certain adult home staff members. However, as we have pointed out, these requirements further obscure the essential nature of adult homes, most of which are incorporated as profit-making, business enterprises. Further, we are critical of the implied notion that such training transforms an adult home into a 'treatment-oriented' supportive environment and staff members into competent and objective mental health workers. We believe these false assumptions will continue to exist as long as the regulations do not explicitly define the relationship between adult home operator and resident as a contractual one. We urge the Department to amend the proposed regulations to clearly reflect such a statement. To do otherwise is to perpetuate an illusion and codify an overt conflict of interest. The operators and staffs of the profit-based adult homes are *not* health care service providers, but are business people providing housing and 'personal care' services in exchange for profit.

If all parties understand the business-contractual nature of the relationship between the adult home operator and residents of such facilities, then it is easy to view residents *not* as 'mental patients' needing treatment, but *rather* as tenants who may or may not choose to avail themselves of the services offered as part of their contractual agreement (admissions agreement). Certainly, not all residents need or may want to use the full array of stipulated services; absolutely no services should be coercively imposed. The role of the regulatory agency then becomes one of ensuring that the services which are contractually offered are of a certain quality, are reflective of the needs of the majority of the people living in such facilities and are not charged to residents' accounts as 'extra services' for which an additional payment is required. We find this operating concept to be very different from the 'treatment team' notion which formed the framework for the existing DAS regulations and which underlies these newly proposed regulations.

We urge the Department to consider this view and to rewrite the regulations so that they reflect the concept of an adult home resident, not as a patient requiring treatment or monitoring, but as a citizen of the community in which she/he resides and who happens *by circumstances* (inability to live alone, no family able to provide housing, etc.) to be living in an adult residential care setting where she/he may or may not need the 'personal care' services which are offered. The criticisms of specific regulations which we present below are based upon this view of adult home residents as quasi-tenants and citizens who, like the rest of us, should be free to choose needed services from an array offered to them by legitimate, not-for-profit service providers.

We want now to address the assumption that in-house case managers, paid by the adult home operators, or case management services provided directly by the operators, can be free from the conflict of interest inherent in the owner-resident relationship. This is an obviously false assumption which fails to recognize that owners' interests are not the same as residents' interests. One of the most important responsibilities of a case manager is advocacy to help ensure that clients receive the full range of stipulated legal rights and entitlements. Many of these rights and entitlements pertain to the operation of the adult home itself and the revenues received. Therefore, the potential for conflict of interest situations in which the 'house' case manager's functions are compromised is self-evident. No matter how 'advocacy-oriented' an operator or operator-employed case manager may be initially, it will not be long before she/he learns the limits that his or her advocacy efforts can take. For example, advocating with SSI to ensure that a resident receive his or her monthly cheque is 'safe' advocacy because both owner and resident benefit; urging that a resident directly challenge the operator and file a former complaint with the regulatory agency if adequate meals are not served is *not* 'safe' advocacy because it involves supporting and encouraging operator-resident conflict and confrontation. Challenging personal allowance policies and practices and confronting an operator when too many people are forced to share a room further illustrates this point.

There is another very important related issue, that of client confidentiality. The newly proposed regulations require that the house-employed case manager be responsible for the coordination of all case management services provided to residents of the home. This is a clear abrogation of clients' rights to confidentiality, unless each individual resident indicates in *writing* that she/he wishes specific information relating to case management services to be shared with the house-employed case manager. Obviously, many residents may not want such information shared, especially if the sharing of such information might put their housing situation in jeopardy. It is important to remember that informed consent is an individual right; it cannot be usurped by a regulation requiring house-employed case managers to perform coordination functions. Regulations must function to protect the rights of all involved parties and care must be taken to ensure that no one party's rights are inadvertently infringed upon.

Case management services targeted toward clients' needs cannot be performed by an adult home operator or an operator-employed case manager. It is imperative that case management functions be performed by individuals employed by outside agencies, whether they be state agencies or voluntary sector, not-for-profit agencies under contract to the Office of Mental Health to provide case management services. Again, we want to stress that the requirement for case management services being made available to adult home residents is a good one; the issue is with how the regulations contradict the intent of these services by legitimating conflict-of-interest in their provision.

We want now to offer comments and criticisms of specific sections of the newly proposed regulations. All of our remarks reflect our perspective on the conceptual framework underlying the regulations, that framework which sees the adult home operator as a mental health 'treatment team' member rather than as a business person whose needs and interests *will necessarily* be different and in conflict with those of the adult home resident.

APPENDIX VI

Problems and Prospects in Mental Patients' Rights

Testimony Prepared By

Stephen M. Rose, Ph.D.
School of Social Welfare – SUNY, Stony Brook

14 March 1978

Publication of a handbook on the rights of psychiatric patients by the Office of Mental Health is certainly a positive step. However, it is also a complex one that involves complicated conceptual issues, problems of delivery of the service, and problems of adequate coverage. I would like to briefly address these three areas of concern.

Conceptual framework

The essential conceptual problem confronting those concerned with 'patients' rights' is this: are people using the services of state psychiatric facilities, who are understood to be in need of psychiatric and other services, to be defined as Citizens who require some form of special attention, or are they to be understood as Mental Patients whose rights constitute some sub-class of citizens? This question must be answered in order to determine whether legal or treatment concerns take priority. But by whom shall the question be answered – psychiatrists or lawyers? The implications of different beginning positions on this question quite obviously lead to different positions of significance. Several examples of this overriding concern appear below:

1 On page 1, the statement is made, 'Any limitation of your rights must be written in your treatment record and must be reviewed periodically.' This

reflects the latter of the two positions identified above – the one which assumes the person to be primarily a Mental Patient rather than a Citizen. The alternative would be to say that 'Any intended limitation of your rights will be reviewed and approved by the Court before being implemented.'

2   On page 2, the statement is made, 'Any limitation on your right to communicate must be explained to you and written in your treatment record.' The alternative would be, 'Any limitation on your right to communicate will be reviewed and approved by a Court before being implemented.'

3   On page 3, the statement is made, 'Anyone interested in you may visit you unless your treatment team, in writing, restricts such visits for medical reasons, or you don't want to see them.' The alternative might be, 'Visitation with you may be done with your permission by any interested person or friend. Should the treatment team feel that this is unadvisable and you disagree, they will restrict visits only after Court review and approval.'

4   As a follow-up to number 3, the statement, 'If agreement is not reached (on visiting), the treatment team may decide on the limitation and enter the reasons for it in the patient's record' is eliminated by the alternative stated above (in number 3).

5   On page 13, under the section on right to object to treatment, the statement is made that in the case of disagreement, 'Treatment may then be started, unless the patient or his representative chooses to appeal the decision to the facility director.' The alternative would be that 'Choices over treatment reside with the person to whom the treatment is to be administered. The reasons for all treatment, and any possible negative effects, including those from medication, must be presented to the person and recorded in the record. Any effort to change this without the approval of the person involved must be reviewed by and approved by a Court.'

When the beginning position on this issue is clear, the reason for a mental patients' rights manual becomes clear. If the person in the hospital is seen as a Citizen, then the reason for the publication and distribution of a manual on patients' rights becomes clear – the rights of people qua Citizens in the hospital have been violated and their beings have been abused by treatment team members, or by other patients because of neglect by treatment team members or insufficient coverage on the unit. In other words, the person is being protected from the hospital. Conversely, if the beginning position on this issue starts with the person redefined as a Mental Patient, then the hospital in the form of treatment team members and others is being protected from legal suit by the patient. This is an irony, since the basis for patients' rights comes out of legal victories won by patients to protect themselves, and the rationale for such rights is not to give patients 'a secure feeling' or to enable them 'to cooperate fully in a treatment program' as is stated in the introduction to the manual. If, in fact, the purpose is to coerce the patient into cooperating with the treatment team, which is the way the document reads, then the introduction should specify that the legal rights described are being listed to inform the patient that he or she is no longer being considered a citizen by the hospital treatment team and will be removed from the legal privileges of citizenship in the manner outlined above in points 1 to 5.

Problems of delivery

Presuming the issues of conceptual framework can be resolved, any manual of rights is going to present difficulties in effective utilization. This has to do with how to implement the plan to use the manual, and this in turn relates to the fact that the document contains complex language which often requires interpretation and discussion. As an example, the opening paragraph in the Introduction on page 1 contains a complete contradiction within it: it says that rights are both 'fully protected' and that 'Other rights may be limited by law or for medical reasons.' Furthermore, with regard to this paragraph, it is confusing to me to figure our how legal rights can be abrogated for medical reasons, when I thought that medical arbitrariness needs to be abrogated by the Law. Other examples include such statements as 'In general, you may send and receive sealed, unopened and uncensored mail'; 'You have a right to receive services from a staff that is competent and is adequate *enough* to administer the service' (p. 8); or 'Drugs may not be used for the convenience of staff . . .' (p. 9), etc. A second problem, of a related nature, is that the document is written and that precludes a large number of people with difficulty in reading from receiving equal benefit which in turn suggests the need for alternative forms of presentation.

Another more complex problem in delivery exists with special reference to people returning to the hospital who had been there for long periods of time on a previous admission. Often in our experience, the lengthy stay in the hospital deprived many of these people of the self-concept or feeling that they are in fact persons qua Citizens, and so they do not often recognize that discussions of legal rights pertain to them. Conveying that such rights do indeed pertain to them is a complex process involving supportive settings and approaches.

Another facet involved is that of evaluation. In order to avoid the situation where discussion of rights becomes a pro forma exercise, an evaluation of effectiveness must be undertaken. In order for any thorough and honest evaluation to be done, the baseline data must come from the patients themselves – e.g., they must be asked what they understand their rights to be rather than whether or not anyone told them about rights in the abstract. And, we would suggest, that such an evaluation be done by either MHIS or, better yet, by an outside body such as the citizens' advisory board to the unit, the ACLU, etc.

With regard to implementation, we also think additional in-service training for staff will be necessary to familiarize them with the legal rights of patients. The scope and nature of this training will of course vary depending upon the orientation taken as discussed above.

Problems of adequate coverage

Everyone learning about their rights as inpatients is at least potentially a candidate for discharge. We urge the Office of Mental Health to prepare a manual covering the rights of people discharged from state hospitals into different settings and to build information about such rights into the discharge process. Our own experience in the Sayville Project after-care program puts us daily into touch with violations of NYS Executive Law 758 – apertaining to residents and owners of private proprietary homes for adults. Patients informed of these rights and how to seek and obtain legal assistance in the community will be in much better position to make a constructive adjustment.

Client Benefit Packet

1 Sayville Project pamphlet – Case Manager and Club dates to be written in. Check for recent Club dates
2 Eligibility Form – OMH 143 (copy to client)
3 Agency Info Form (copy to client)
4 OMH Release Form – OMH 144 (copy to client)
5 Handicapped ID Form and pamphlet
6 Bus Routes
7 Medicaid Transportation. Cab will transport when called. Check for current update. Cab numbers: Commercial Taxi – Medford 698–8222 Town Taxi – E. Islip 581–4477, 112 Taxi – Patchogue 475–6213
8 Adult Home or SRO booklet
9 Voter registration – list of legislators

SAYVILLE PROJECT
Community Support Systems Programme
Case Manager Contact Sheet

Client Contact ☐

Inter-organizational ☐
Contact

Client: Date:

Residence: Staff:

Agency involved/Agency Staff:

List issues discussed:

Process summary:

Follow-up Plan (if applicable):

SUSB 2148-01 R-2 F122 [8-82]

Bibliography

Allen, Priscella, 'A Consumer's View of California's Mental Health Care System,' *Psychiatric Quarterly*, 48 (1974), pp. 1–13.

Avirim, U. and Segal, S.P., 'Exclusion of the Mentally Ill: Reflection of an Old Problem in a New Context,' *Archives of General Psychiatry*, 29 (July 1973), pp. 126–31.

Bachrach, Leona L., 'Deinstitutionalization: An Analytical Review and Sociological Perspective,' *Mental Health Statistical Series D*, No. 4, Rockville, Md.: NIMH, 1976.

Bachrach, Leona L., 'Deinstitutionalization: A Conceptual Framework,' Rockville, Md.: NIMH, 1977.

Bassuk, Ellen L. and Gerson, Samuel, 'Deinstitutionalization and Mental Health Services,' *Scientific American*, Vol. 238, No.2 (February 1978).

Baxter, Ellen and Hopper, Kim, *Private Lives/Public Spaces: Homeless Adults on the Streets of New York City*, New York: Community Service Society Institute for Welfare Research, 1981.

Berger, Peter and Luckmann, Thomas, *The Social Construction of Reality*, Garden City, N.Y.: Anchor, 1967.

Black, Bruce L, *The Myth of Deinstitutionalization: Inter-organizational Maintenance of the Medical Model in the Community*, unpublished Ph.D. Dissertation, State University of New York at Stony Brook, 1982.

Brenner, M.H., *Mental Illness and the Economy*, Cambridge, Mass.: Harvard University Press, 1973.

Campbell, Donald, 'Reforms as Experiments,' *American Psychologist*, 24 (April 1969), pp. 409–29.

Chu, F.D. and Trotter, S., *The Madness Establishment: Ralph Nader's Group Report on the National Institute of Mental Health*, New York: Grossman, 1974.

Comptroller General of the United States, *Returning the Mentally Disabled to the Community: Government Needs to Do More*, Washington, D.C.: Government Accounting Office, 1977.

Conrad, Peter and Schneider, J.W., *Deviance and Medicalization: From Badness to Sickness*, St Louis: C.U. Mosby Co., 1980.

Cox, Judith F., 'Executive Summary of Policies and Guidelines for Core Service Agencies and Case Management Programs,' New York State Office of Mental Health (April 1981).

Estroff, Sue E., *Making it Crazy*, Berkeley: University of California Press, 1981.

Freire, Paolo, *Pedagogy of the Oppressed*, New York: The Seabury Press, 1968.

Freire, Paolo, *Education for Critical Consciousness*, New York: The Seabury Press, 1973.

Goffman, Erving, *Asylums: Essays on the Social Situation of Mental Patients and Other Inmates*, Garden City: Doubleday Anchor Books, 1961.

Gouldner, Alvin, *The Coming Crisis of Western Sociology*, New York: Basic Books, 1970.

Hudson, Barclay, 'Domains of Evaluation,' *Social Policy*, September/October 1975.

Hyman, Herbert, *Survey Design and Analysis*, New York: The Free Press of Glencoe, 1955.

Hyman, Herbert *et al.*, *Interviewing in Social Research*, Chicago: University of Chicago Press, 1954.

Hynes, C.J., *Private Proprietary Homes for Adults: An Interim Report*, New York State Deputy Attorney General's Office, 1977.

Johnson, Diane M., Taichman, Ettie and Rose, Stephen, M., '*You Catch More Flies with Honey than with Vinegar': A Follow-Up Study of Legal Rights Training for Mental Health Workers in Suffolk County, New York*, Mental Health Project, Stony Brook, 1982 (mimeographed).

Joint Commission on Mental Illness and Health, *Action for Mental Health*, New York: Basic Books, 1961.

Klerman, G., 'Current Evaluation Research on Mental Health Sciences,' *American Journal of Psychiatry*, 131 (1974), pp. 783–8.

Kuhn, Thomas S., *The Structure of Scientific Revolutions*, Chicago: University of Chicago Press, 1962.

Lander, Louise, 'The Mental Health Con Game,' *Health/Pac Bulletin*, No. 65 (July/August 1975).

Lehman, D.W., 'Abuse Begins at Home: Inside the Adult Home Business,' *Village Voice* (3 September 1979), 1, pp. 24–5.

Long, Norton, 'The Local Community as an Ecology of Games,' in *The Polity* (Long, Norton), Chicago: Rand McNally and Co., 1962.

Marcuse, Herbert, *One Dimensional Man*, Boston: Beacon Press, 1964.

Mental Health Law Project, *Project Summary: July 1979 – June 1981*, Washington, D.C., 1981.

Mills, C.W., *The Sociological Imagination*, New York: Oxford University Press, 1959.

Morrissey, J.P., Hall, Richard H. and Lindsey, Michael, *Interorganizational Relations: A Sourcebook of Measures for Mental Health Programs*, Rockville, Md.: NIMH, 1981.

Nachimus, D., *Public Policy Evaluation*, New York: St Martin's Press, 1979.

Navarro, Vincente, 'Health and the Corporate Society', *Social Policy*, Jan/Feb, 1975.

Navarro, Vicente, 'Work, Ideology and Science: The Case of Medicine', in Vicente Navarro and Daniel M. Berman (eds), *Health and Work under Capitalism: An International Perspective*, Farmingdale, N.Y.: Baywood Publishing Co., Inc. 1983.

New York State Assembly Joint Committee to Study the Department of Mental Hygiene, *Mental Health in New York*, Albany: New York State Assembly, 1976.

New York State Legislative Commission on Expenditure Review, *Patients Released from State Psychiatric Centers*, Albany, N.Y., 1975.

New York State Office of Mental Health, *Five Year Comprehensive Plan for Mental Health Services*, Albany, N.Y., 1981.

New York State Senate Mental Hygiene and Addiction Control Committee, *Single Room Occupancy Hotels: A Dead End in the Human Services Delivery System*, Albany, N.Y., 1980.

New York State Senate Minority Task Force on Deinstitutionalization, *Mental Disorder: The Deinstitutionalization Problem in New York State*, Albany, N.Y., 1979.

O'Conner, James, *The Fiscal Crisis of the State*, New York: St Martin's Press, 1973.

Panzetta, A.F., *Community Mental Health: Myth and Reality*, Philadelphia: Lea and Febiger, 1971.

Perrow, Charles, 'The Analysis of Goals in Complex Organizations,' *American Sociological Review*, Vol. 26, No. 6 (December 1961).

Perrow, Charles, 'Demystifying Organizations,' in *The Management of Human Services*, in R.C. Sarri and Y. Hasenfeld (eds), New York: Columbia University Press, 1978.

Pfeffer, Jeffrey and Salancik, Gerald, R., *The External Control of Organizations*, New York: Harper & Row, 1978.

President's Commission on Mental Health, *Report and Recommendations to the President, Vol. I*, Washington D.C., Superintendent of Documents, U.S. Government Printing Office, 1978.

Prevost, James, A., M.D., *Deinstitutionalization in New York State: Mental Health Programs, Progress and Plans* (A Progress Report to Governor Hugh L. Carey), New York State Office of Mental Heath, Albany, N.Y., 1978.

Rose, Stephen M., *Betrayal of the Poor: The Transformation of Community Action*, Cambridge, Mass.: Schenkman, 1972.

Rose, Stephen M., 'After-Care Rights and Responsibilities,' unpublished, State University of New York at Stony Brook, 1977a.

Rose, Stephen M., 'Contradictions in Deinstitutionalization Policy and Program: Comments and Recommendations on After-Care'. Testimony for New York State Assembly Subcommittee on After-Care, unpublished, State University of New York at Stony Brook, 1977b.

Rose, Stephen M., 'Misjudgment in the New Era: Continuity in the Treatment of Those Called Mentally Ill,' unpublished, State University of New York at Stony Brook, 1977c.

Rose, Stephen, M., 'The Transformation of Community Action,' in *New Perspectives on the American Community: A Book of Readings,* third ed, (ed. Warren, Roland), Chicago: Rand McNally, 1977d.

Rose, Stephen M., 'Adult Protective Services: C.A.S.A. Policy Paper,' Community After-Care Service Association, unpublished, Sayville, N.Y., 1978a.

Rose, Stephen, M., 'Deinstitutionalization – A Challenge to the Profession,' Paper delivered for the Institute on Deinstitutionalization at the National Conference on Social Welfare, Los Angeles, Ca., 1978b.

Rose, Stephen M. and Chaglasian, Donna, 'Discharged Mental Patients,' *The Social Welfare Forum, 1978*, Columbia University Press, 1978.

Rosenhan, D.L., 'On Being Sane in Insane Places,' *Science*, Vol. 179 (January 1973).

Rossi, P.H., Freeman, H.E. and Wright, S.R., *Evaluation: A Systematic Approach*, Beverly Hills, Ca.: Sage Publications, 1979.

Ryan, William, *Blaming the Victim*, revised, updated edn, New York: Vintage Books, 1976.

Reinhardt, Uwe E., 'Proposed Changes in the Organization of Health-Care Delivery: An Overview and Critiques, *Milbank Memorial Fund Quarterly*, 51 (Spring 1973), pp. 169–222.

Scott, W. Richard, 'Effectiveness of Organizational Effectiveness Studies,' in *New Perspectives on Organizational Effectiveness* pp. 63–95 in Paul S. Goodman and Johannes M. Pennings, (eds), San Francisco: Jossey-Bass, 1977.

Scott, W. Richard, *Organizations: Rational, Natural, and Open Systems*, Englewood Cliffs, N.J.: Prentice-Hall, 1981.

Scull, Andrew, *Decarceration: Community Treatment and the Deviant – A Radical View*, Englewood Cliffs, N.J.: Prentice-Hall, 1977.

Sennett, Richard and Cobb, Jonathan, *Hidden Injuries of Class*, New York: Vintage Books, 1973.

Steindorff, S., 'Implementing Community Support Systems in a Turbulent Environment: Building on Quicksand,' New York State Office of Mental Health (February 1979).

Taichman, Ettie and Ellaborn, Diane, *Your Legal Rights as an Adult Home Resident*, Mental Health Project, School of Social Welfare, State University of New York at Stony Brook, 1980a.

Taichman, Ettie, Careccia, Gerry and Bishop, Hal, *Your Legal Rights When you Rent a Room*, Mental Health Project, School of Social Welfare, State University of New York at Stony Brook, 1980b.

Taichman, Ettie, Johnson, D., Keelty, M. and Schaefer, L., 'The Rental Agreement: A Legislative Proposal for S.R.O.'s,' mimeographed, The Mental Health Project, School of Social Welfare, State University of New York at Stony Brook, 1980c.

Turner, J.C. and TenHoor, W.J., 'The N.I.M.H. Community Support Program: Pilot Approach to a Needed Social Reform,' *Schizophrenic Bulletin*, Vol. 4, No. 3, 1978.

Van Nieuwenhuijze, C.A.O., *Society As Process*, The Hague: Mouton and Company, 1962.

Warren, Roland L., *The Community in America*, Chicago: Rand McNally College Publishing Co., 1963.

Warren, Roland L., 'The Interorganizational Field as a Focus for Investigation,' *Administrative Science Quarterly*, 12, No. 3 (December 1967).

Warren Roland L., 'The Sociology of Knowledge and the Problems of the Inner Cities,' in *New Perspectives on the American Community: A Book of Readings* (ed. Warren, R.L.), third edn, Chicago: Rand McNally College Publishing Co., 1977.

Warren, Roland L., Rose, Stephen and Bergunder, Ann, *The Structure of Urban Reform*, Lexington, Mass.: D.C. Heath and Co., 1974.

Weiss, Carol H. (ed.), *Evaluating Action Programs: Readings in Social Action and Education*, Boston, Mass.: Allyn & Bacon, Inc., 1972.